"The keys to the kingdom! A leading Erickson scholar plus two of the master's daughters describe the core strategies and techniques that underlie his legacy of healing and therapeutic utilization of clients' resources. This brilliant book is a 'must-read' for anyone interested in understanding and applying Erickson's work. Highly recommended!"

Michael F. Hoyt, PhD
Author of *Some Stories are Better than Others, Interviews with Brief Therapy Experts,* **and** *The Present is a Gift*

"In this engaging book renowned experts, Dan Short, Betty Alice Erickson, and Roxanna Erickson Klein, shed new light on fundamental patterns in the work of Milton H. Erickson, MD. Immerse yourself deeply in this entrancing and timeless wisdom, and realize the power within."

Jeffrey K. Zeig, PhD
Author of *Teaching Seminar with Milton H. Erickson, MD* **and** *Experiencing Erickson*

"As the era of well-meaning, but misguided victimology wanes, psycho-therapists are rediscovering the hope and resiliency that permeate the timeless therapeutic strategies of Milton H. Erickson. The authors, family and insiders who know Dr. Erickson best, lucidly and impressively convey new insights into the philosophy of healing that is at the core of his psychotherapeutic genius. By understanding that healing is the activation of inner resources during the process of recovery, making life a continuous process of rehabilitation, psychotherapists can markedly improve their therapeutic effectiveness and bring new hope to their patients."

Nicholas A. Cummings, PhD, ScD
Author of *Focused Psychotherapy* **and** *The Essence of Psychotherapy*

"In this age of standardized and even manualized treatments, *Hope & Resiliency* provides a refreshing reminder about the importance of honoring each individual's uniqueness. The authors build on the creative and highly skilled work of Milton Erickson and do a wonderful job of making some aspects of his methods more accessible to the reader. The case examples and family stories bring a folksy charm and gentle wisdom to the authors' clinically astute considerations of what it takes to do therapy well."

Michael D. Yapko, PhD
Author of *Trancework* **and** *Treating Depression With Hypnosis*

"This is a delightful introduction to the work of Milton Erickson. It is remarkably clear and chalk full of practical examples and applications. It is especially good at emphasizing Erickson's positive and remarkably creative way of accepting and utilizing all parts of a person's reality to allow significant change and growth. I look forward to recommending it to my students as essential reading."

Author of *Therapeutic Trances, The*

"Hope & Resiliency is a delightful and deeply moving reading experience that facilitated peace and well-being within my own heart and mind. I will keep it by my bedside as a daily refresher in the healing legacy Milton H. Erickson has passed on to all of us."

Ernest L. Rossi, PhD
Author of *The Psychobiology of Gene Expression*

"A must-read for every therapist. The book combines clear, simple instructions with wonderful case studies and an emphasis on Erickson's belief in the inner strength and the unlimited potential of each individual. The family anecdotes are precious."

Cloé Madanes
Author of *Behind The One-Way Mirror, Sex, Love & Violence*
and *Strategic Family Therapy*

"Another welcome addition describing the wisdom of Milton H. Erickson, MD by three authors who know his work well. This book makes a connection between his personal and professional life and presents detailed clinical examples for therapists in the field."

Jay Haley, MA
Author of *Uncommon Therapy, Art of Strategic Therapy, Ordeal Therapy* **and**
Problem Solving Therapy

"Hope & Resiliency: Understanding the Psychotherapeutic Strategies of Milton H. Erickson, MD is a wonderful book. I had the sense while reading it that I was in Erickson's office and just listening to him talk. This is a consequence of an informal narrative style wherein the book contains many case studies, comments by Erickson, and comments by his daughters and Short. I have not seen some of these studies and commentaries before, and they shed a new and continuingly interesting light on this remarkable man and his works. There are gems like, 'Let patients know that they *are* going to be cured and that it will take place *within* them' and 'Often in psychotherapy a change of reference is all that is needed' and 'Erickson's philosophy of healing was characterized by his *attention* to the goodness of the patient's mind and body.'

"The heart of the book centers around organizing Erickson's contributions under the categories of: distraction, partitioning, progression, suggestion, reorientation, and utilization. Although it is next to impossible to characterize or systematize Erickson's work in simple packets, this organization does lend itself to a useful set of guidelines to the man and his work.

"This book is highly recommended as it provides the reader with some unique perspectives on Erickson's work, his way of working, and many practical ideas."

Rubin Battino, MS
Author of *Metaphoria, Guided Imagery and Other Approaches to Healing*
and *Ericksonian Approaches*

Hope & Resiliency
Understanding the Psychotherapeutic Strategies of Milton H. Erickson, MD

Dan Short, PhD
Betty Alice Erickson, MS, LPC
Roxanna Erickson-Klein, RN, PhD

**Foreword by
Stephen Lankton, MSW, DAHB**

Crown House Publishing Limited
www.crownhouse.co.uk
www.crownhousepublishing.com

First published by
Crown House Publishing Ltd
Crown Buildings, Bancyfelin, Carmarthen, Wales, SA33 5ND, UK
www.crownhouse.co.uk

and

Crown House Publishing Company LLC
PO Box 2223, Williston, VT 05495
www.crownhousepublishing.com

British Library Cataloguing-in-Publication Data
A catalogue entry for this book is available
from the British Library.

Hardback ISBN 978-190442493-2
Paperback ISBN 978-178583158-4
Mobi ISBN 978-184590255-1
ePub ISBN 978-184590613-9

LCCN 2005924702

In the desert of Sonora, on the branch of a tree,
Sat a noble eagle gazing to sea.
Wings forged from iron, a shadow was sown
Within was the hope of dreams not yet known.

Eagle readied for flight looking far and away.
Tree branch grew light, the shadow did stay
A journey of discovery into the sun;
The shadow, the eagle and the tree are one.

By Roxanna Erickson-Klein

The eagle pictured on the cover is from Milton Erickson's extensive collection of Seri Indian ironwood carvings. Carved from hidden roots that are centuries old, these Indian artifacts allegedly bring good fortune and long life. It seems only appropriate that this unique material—wood that does not float—would serve as an icon for a man who continues to defy static categorization.

Acknowledgments

This book draws on the knowledge of other authors and leaders in the field and to each of them we express our gratitude for helping light the way on our journey of discovery. We thank Jeff Zeig and Jay Haley for providing expert feedback during the initial development of the manuscript. Valuable critiques were also provided by Consuelo Casula and Claudia Weinspach who helped prepare the way for international distribution. Dan Short is especially grateful to Teresa Robles who provided the initial encouragement to write the book.

Also, many thanks from each of us to the publishing team at Crown House for having enough faith and enthusiasm in the project to make the book be as good as it can be.

Contents

Foreword

At the time of his death on March 25, 1980, Milton H. Erickson, MD was said to have written over 300 professional papers and hypnotized over 30,000 subjects. Today, there are 118 Institutes established worldwide for the further study and practice of Erickson's contributions to hypnosis, brief therapy, family therapy and psychotherapy. A search on the Internet today reveals over 78,000 entries under his name. Amazon.com lists 132 books in a search for his name. Even eBay has items for sale pertaining to Dr Erickson! With all this effort to explain the work of Dr Erickson, I still find that *Hope & Resiliency* is a breath of fresh air.

Erickson's work has grown from a seed to a forest over the last few decades. This is in large part due to the tireless work of Dr Jeffrey Zeig, Director of the Milton H. Erickson Foundation, Inc. in Phoenix, Arizona as well as the many dedicated faculty members who teach at the Foundation's training events.

Over the years Erickson's work became increasingly refined. In fact, early visitors to his office often disagreed about his approach when speaking to those of us who visited him in later years. The reason for this is obvious if we trace the progression of Dr Erickson's work over the years from Eloise to Phoenix. We can look at the duration of his treatment, the use of suggestion from direct to indirection, at least, during the induction process (if not for treatment also). Also, we could trace the progression in the use of therapeutic metaphors and brief therapy. Additionally, let's consider some changes in the view of symptoms from a psychoanalytic view to an interactional view. This latter will show a change in viewing people and problems which quite logically goes hand in hand with the above.

Treatment Duration

In the early 1950s we see several cases over which Erickson took several months. The case of the man with a 'fat lip' took upwards of 11 months (Erickson and Rossi, 1979) and the case of the "February Man" from Michigan took far longer – up to 2 years (Erickson, 1980). While it is true that Dr Erickson made himself available to clients for an indefinite period of time while he lived in Phoenix, his published cases became shorter in duration. In 1973 we find the case of the 8 year old 'stomper' which took 2 hours (Haley, 1973). Various cases of his "shock" technique in 1973 entailed 1 to 2 hour long sessions (Erickson and Rossi, 1980). In general, the movement to brief therapy progressed continually and became prominent in his practice in the late 1970s and beyond.

Hypnotic Suggestion

In a 1957 transcript of induction, we find Dr Erickson's redundant use of words like "sleep" as in the following quote, "Now I want you to *go deeper and deeper asleep*" (Haley, 1967). In addition his authoritative approach can be found in this same transcript represented with the statement "*I can put you* in any level of trance" [italics mine] " (Haley, 1967). However, by 1976 Erickson believed indirect suggestion to be a "significant factor" in his work (Erickson, Rossi et al., 1976, p. 452). Furthermore, by 1981 Erickson clearly states that he "offers" ideas and suggestions (Erickson and Rossi, 1981, pp. 1–2) and explicitly adds, "I don't like this matter of telling a patient *I want you to get tired and sleepy*" (Erickson and Rossi, 1981, p. 4) [italics mine]. With regard to his use of indirect approaches, there is clear evidence that Erickson's practice evolved to a point in the late 1970s where he had abandoned his earlier techniques of redundancy and authoritarianism during induction.

The Use of Metaphor as Indirect Intervention

In 1944 Erickson reluctantly published "The Method Employed to Formulate a Complex Story for the Induction of the Experimental Neurosis" (Haley, 1967). His understanding at that point was that a complex story that paralleled a client's problem could actually heighten the client's discomfort and bring the neurosis closer to the surface. Within a decade, in 1954, Erickson was using many "fabricated case histories" of fleeting symptomatology (Erickson,

1980). Still, almost two decades later in 1973, we see that Erickson provides several examples of case stories for making a therapeutic point (Haley, 1973) and by 1979 Erickson and Rossi actually use the heading of "Metaphor" as a class of interventions (Erickson and Rossi, 1979). Again, this movement corresponds to his movement from direct and authoritarian therapy to indirect and permissive therapy.

Erickson's Conceptualization of Symptoms

From his earliest years as a psychiatrist at least up to 1954, Erickson took a traditional analytic view of neurosis and various symptoms. He said the development of neurotic symptoms "constitutes behavior of a defensive, protective character" (Erickson, 1980). By the mid-1960s his view had become much more interactional. Perhaps this was a result of his collaboration with Jay Haley, Gregory Bateson, John Weakland and the Palo Alto Communication Project. In any case Erickson writes, in 1966, "Mental disease is the breaking down of communication between people" (Erickson, 1980). However, by the end of his career he had moved even further from the analytic and the communications/ systems theory of disease. He states that, symptoms are "forms of communication" and "cues of developmental problems that are in the process of becoming conscious" (Erickson and Rossi, 1979). In summary, the evolution of thought concerning the nature of problems became less oriented to a pathological explanation until, in the end, symptoms could be seen as communication signals of desired directions of growth. Erickson took such signals to be a request for change, and even unconscious contracts for therapeutic engagement.

Cure Accomplished by Reassociation of Experience not Direct Suggestion

The one area in which Erickson never wavered was his view of "cure." I suspect this was a result of his personal experience overcoming paralysis. He learned as a young adult that experiential resources created change. As early as 1948 Erickson recognized that cure was not the result of direct suggestion that somehow influenced the client but was due to the reassociation of experiences that were needed in a particular problematic context (Erickson, 1980). In the later years of his career we find this theme repeated again and again (Erickson and Rossi, 1979; Erickson and Rossi, 1980; Erickson and Rossi, 1981).

Dr Erickson's own explanations were often frustrating to many of us, as he insisted upon sharing wisdom in a rather folksy manner. For instance, asked what the most important thing was in therapy, he would comment, "Speak the client's own experiential language." When asked for the next most important thing to do he commented, "Put one foot in the client's world and leave one foot in your own." Such comments seemed to side step conventional scientific language and left one wondering if he would eventually come to add more. He never would. The many books that have been written about his work often attempt to rectify this situation. The authors quote Rogers, Bandura, hypnosis research, Berne, Szasz, Perls and many others to connect existing knowledge to Erickson's folksy wisdom.

Enter *Hope & Resiliency*. This is a superb book by Dan Short, Betty Alice Erickson, and Roxanna Erickson Klein who have retained Erickson's own words and yet still manage to paint a powerful, comprehensive, and extremely workable theoretical structure. They have created a well-woven theoretical discussion that is a breath of fresh air for those who are ready for an approach based on principles of engagement and change rather than mechanization. *Hope & Resiliency* is not a micro-analysis of techniques, nor should it be. A solid text of Erickson's work needs to highlight the functional principles of how change happens yet still provide comprehensible links to practical interventions. This is exactly what this book does.

Part I introduces Erickson's philosophical foundations. It presents several cases to clearly illustrate the therapist's job as a catalyst for change. Above all, the therapist must respect the wisdom of the client's unconscious and help the client appreciate the same. The best way to accomplish that is through mutual discovery with the client.

Part II presents six key clinical strategies that can provide the foundation for all interventions using an Ericksonian approach. With these six strategies or principles, the authors almost completely circumscribe the vast range of approaches taken by Dr Erickson.

In each situation the authors present strategies in great detail to ensure deep understanding. Specific interventions are not given because the concept of the book is to suggest the strategies from which uncountable creative interventions might be born. As in Part I, each section of the book provides case illustrations and Erickson's actual words to illustrate the points of concern. The authors discuss the strategies of distraction, partitioning, progression, suggestion, reorientation, and utilization. Here is a brief summary to set the stage for the author's detailed case discussions and interpretations.

Distraction pertains to the logic of helping the client break the attention given to experiences that lead to failure. Self-fulfilling prophecies and self-defeating behavior are the best examples.

Partitioning is a strategy for re-chunking or re-parsing the client's problems, goals, resources, attention, and even time and space.

Progression is a matter of building ever increasing gains from small beginnings. The authors give us several new ways to think about progression including geometric, progressive, cognitive, disruptive, and time oriented.

Suggestion is the most significant section for me as I believe suggestion to be foundational to both therapy and socialization. From the authors' vantage point, the use of suggestion, as exemplified by Erickson, becomes a seminal concept as it underlies not just therapy, but also communication in everyday life. The authors explain the connection between the apparent polarities of therapy and daily living as these relate to suggestion. They help readers understand how therapeutic ideas are conveyed both in and out of formal therapy.

Reorientation is a strategy the authors consider one of the most pervasive in therapy. They describe how each new idea introduced to a client should be formulated for a future success or use and how the job of therapy is to continually create this future associational link. They relate this concept to the work of Victor Frankl and Pat Love, the reframing and externalization carried out in Gestalt therapy, Satir sculpting, and psychodrama. Time distortion is described as a major tool for reorientation.

Utilization is the most distinctive strategy in the book as it was one of the hallmarks of Erickson's work in his opinion. Utilization is a process of using the client's energy, point of view, skills, and potentials. The aim is acceptance and motivation of the client to support the distraction, progression, and reorientation. Of course, as clients' behavior is utilized for their own growth, a sense of hope and confidence is automatically instilled. Finally, *Hope & Resiliency* provides a wonderful appendix for learning each of the strategies in the reader's own life and therapy practice.

Dr Dan Short did an unprecedented thing in the preparation of this book. After the initial compilation of this material, the framework, or draft, was shown to colleagues in a dozen different countries around the world. Dr Short collaborated with several other well-known practitioners of Dr Erickson's work so that they might take his basic draft and write adaptations of the work. Thus, he created a cluster of books, each reflecting a differing cultural milieu world-wide. Each version became an adaptation in which the local co-authors modified and tailored the contents of this book to address culturally specific ideas and concepts. *Hope & Resiliency* has thus been transformed, by the addition of indigenous literature and culturally relevant anecdotes, into a work that is specific to each culture in which it was co-authored. The broad scope of this project to write *Hope & Resiliency*, is therefore not limited by the personal experiences of the original authors, but rather represents the combined resources of a large number of highly talented multi-national individuals, and reflects the differing circumstances and ideas of people around the world. I believe this is the first time such a project has ever been created in this manner … and it is a brilliant idea. The global scope of the project for *Hope & Resiliency* may be a unique and original model for the very future of clinical collaboration. If it should turn out to be so, it would be another facet of Dr Erickson's fundamental principles. It truly allows every to speak in their own language around the world; it co-creates rather than dictates.

In the perennial conflict between researchers and clinicians, the voice of those professionals who repeatedly create change in their clients always leads the way. Now, with the world-wide publication of *Hope & Resiliency*, that voice becomes a global baseline for a deeper understanding and development of successful methods of change promoted by Dr Erickson.

In conclusion, an important and often overlooked concept in Erickson's approach is not only *not* ignored here, but it is part of the very fabric of this project on a global level. There has never been a part of Erickson's work that was intended to manipulate or trick a client. Of course, all change-agents are capable of influencing others. That aspect of intervention is all too often the subject of modern clinical works. Further, in the case of change like that accomplished by Dr Erickson, it is all too easy to discuss and elaborate the types of manipulations that lead to change rather than get to the heart of the matter of psychotherapy. This book does not attempt to capitalize on that obvious and easily misunderstood and misinterpreted aspect of interpersonal influence. Instead, the principles behind Erickson's work are shown here to enhance, enrich, and empower each individual in a unique and personal way. Since they are not meant to manipulate or coerce, they are not developed or discussed in that light. *Hope & Resiliency* shows a deep respect for this potential problem. At all times it is about enriching and empowering clients, and helping therapists establish a framework or two to do the same in a myriad of unique ways that matches the myriad of unique clients. What a delightful book this is for introducing refreshing schemes for therapy taken from Erickson's own words and cased and delivered by Dr Short, and two of Erickson's professionally accredited children—psychotherapist Betty Alice Erickson, MBS, LPC and Roxanna Erickson-Klein, RN, PhD.

Stephen Lankton, MSW, DAHB

Editor, American Journal of Clinical Hypnosis, Past-President, Diplomate, American Hypnosis Board for Clinical Social Work

References

Erickson, M. (1980). February Man: Facilitating New Identity in Hypnotherapy. *The collected papers of Milton H.: Erickson on hypnosis: Vol. 4. Innovative hypnotherapy*. E. L. Rossi. New York, Irvington: 525–542.

Erickson, M. (1980b). Method Employed to Formulate a Complex Story for the Induction of an Experimental Neurosis in a Hypnotic Subject. The collected papers of Milton H. Erickson on hypnosis: Vol. 3. Hypnotic investigation of psychodynamic processes. E. L. Rossi (Ed.). New York, Irvington: 336–355.

Erickson, M. (1980). Hypnotic Psychotherapy. *The collected papers of Milton H.: Erickson on hypnosis: Vol. 4. Innovative hypnotherapy*. E. L. Rossi. New York, Irvington: 35–48.

Erickson, M. (1980). Hypnosis: It's Renaissance as a Treatment Modality. *The collected papers of Milton H.: Erickson on hypnosis: Vol. 4. Innovative hypnotherapy*. E. L. Rossi. New York, Irvington: 3–75.

Erickson, M. (1980). Special Techniques of Brief Hypnotherapy. *The collected papers of Milton H.: Erickson on hypnosis: Vol. 4. Innovative hypnotherapy*. E. L. Rossi. New York, Irvington: 149–187.

Erickson, M. and E. Rossi (1979). *Hypnotherapy: An exploratory casebook*. New York, Irvington.

Erickson, M. and E. Rossi (1980). Indirect Forms of Suggestion. *The collected papers of Milton H.: Erickson on hypnosis: Vol. 1 The nature of hypnosis and suggestion*. E. L. Rossi. New York, Irvington: 452–477.

Erickson, M. and E. L. Rossi (1980). Two Level Communication and the Micro Dynamics of Trance and Suggestion. *The collected papers of Milton H. Erickson on hypnosis: Vol. 1 The nature of hypnosis and suggestion*. E. L. Rossi. New York, Irvington: 430–451.

Erickson, M. and E. Rossi (1981). *Experiencing hypnosis: Therapeutic approaches to altered state*. New York, Irvington.

Erickson, M. H., E. L. Rossi, et al. (1976). *Hypnotic realities: The induction of clinical hypnosis and forms of indirect suggest*. New York, Irvington.

Haley, J. (1967). *Advanced techniques of hypnosis and therapy: Selected papers of Milton H. Erickson, M.D.* New York, Grune & Stratton.

Haley, J. (1973). *Uncommon therapy: The psychiatric techniques of Milton H. Erickson, M.D.* New York, Norton.

Preface

Contained within these pages is an account of health-oriented problem-solving that provides a clear, useful guide for responding to those who are seeking help. Such hardships include psychopathology, chronic medical conditions, family dysfunction, addiction, trauma, academic delay, social failure, and other distressing or demoralizing circumstances. The application of these strategies is unusually broad because the underlying concepts provide access to the core of human problem solving.

In every instance of family, organizational, or cultural progress, the fundamental unit of change is the individual. Hope and resiliency provides a path toward whatever good the future may hold. Without having sufficient hope or resiliency, vast amounts of external resources can be poured into what is essentially a vacuum of despair and surrender. People who are persuaded to believe in themselves put forth greater effort, which increases the probability of success (Bandura, 2003). This focus on hope and resiliency is consistent with the positive psychology movement that has emerged within mainstream psychology and it is a useful way to conceptualize the pioneering work of Milton H. Erickson.

The psychotherapeutic approach of Dr Erickson is considered by many to be the work of a genius, but his methodology is sometimes difficult to understand. Erickson's most celebrated clinical cases have in common a seemingly insurmountable problem that is elegantly resolved through a surprisingly simple and resourceful solution. Under careful examination, the subtle nuances and complexities of his techniques are daunting. Yet, for Erickson, the interventions were natural behaviors derived from commonsense reasoning. The question we are confronted with is *how* this type of remarkable clinical intuition can be learned.

Many efforts to learn Erickson's approach to psychotherapy have focused on identifying and replicating his techniques. Much of the Ericksonian literature provides microdynamic analyses of Erickson's words and actions so that these behaviors can be imitated. The importance of these works and of studying Erickson's numerous innovative techniques is not to be underestimated. By studying the artistry of Milton Erickson, a greater appreciation for his skill is developed.

"There is," as Erickson stated, "a tremendous need to utilize … an awareness of techniques and an awareness of the kinds of techniques that you as an individual can employ" (Erickson, 1959a).

Although a study of techniques is a good starting point, when a practitioner's education is restricted to learning technical procedures there is a tendency to develop the mistaken assumption that therapy is something that must be "done to" the patient.[1] In contrast, there is a great deal of research which suggests that technique accounts for only a minor portion of the measurable positive outcomes in psychotherapy (Duncan, Miller, and Sparks, 2004). While continually adding to one's repertoire of techniques, it is essential to recognize the broader concepts of transformation that make change possible. As will be discussed later, unless the inner resources of the patient are recognized and engaged, even the best techniques will fail. Only with a broad and well-grounded appreciation of the process of healing and growth will a therapist's clinical judgment be sound.

Another problem with seeking to replicate Erickson's work is that the specific interventions he used are not always appropriate in today's world. Much of the casework used to illustrate the concepts in this text is drawn from Erickson's work during the 1930s through the 1960s. While looking for timeless lessons, the context of the time, the milieu, and societal resources must also be considered.

---

[1] In recent times, the term "patient" has become highly politicized. Some automatically assume that its use implies a superior role for the helper with the helpee stuck in the position of inferior. Others, such as Nicholas Cummings, have argued that the term implies equality among the various branches of healthcare. Because Erickson identified the people he worked with as "patients," in all of his writings and lectures, we have made similar use of the term. Erickson is quoted frequently in this book so the decision was made to favor continuity and clarity rather than becoming embroiled in an argument over political correctness.

The resources and goals of society have changed dramatically from when Erickson practiced. During the first three decades of Erickson's career, mental hospitals housed a large percentage of individuals who could not adapt to independent living. In contemporary practice there is a focus on the "least invasive" intervention with many new resources such as hot lines, halfway houses, and the vast expansion of Social Security disability payments and Medicaid for people who have physical and psychological disabilities. Furthermore, in Erickson's time there were few psychotropic drugs available, and most that were available had debilitating and devastating side effects. Recent discoveries in the biochemical realm have created new opportunities for helping individuals with chronic mental illness.

Furthermore, Erickson's integration of personal life with professional practice is nearly impossible to replicate in today's urban society. There are new standards of accountability, limitations and boundary definitions that were not present at the time Erickson practiced. Although his emphasis on building alliances will never become outdated, some of his methods are no longer considered to be socially or professionally correct. It is both unrealistic and undesirable for clinicians today to practice exactly as Erickson did.

Students of any field require a certain amount of structured knowledge in order to benefit from the experiences of those who came before them. However, throughout history, human progress has been impeded by the problem of blind repetition and orthodoxy. New innovations are not possible when the specialists of any field confine themselves to step-by-step procedures for conducting their craft. The same is certainly true for psychotherapy. We stand on the shoulders of those who came before us not by working from the mold that they cast but by recognizing the function of their design. It is with this spirit of innovation that we will begin our journey of discovery guided by the psychotherapeutic strategies of Milton H. Erickson, MD.

A Biographical Sketch of Milton H. Erickson

Overview

For Milton H. Erickson (1901–80), hope and resiliency were a way of living life and therefore a natural basis for his approach to psychotherapy. Erickson began practicing medicine in the late 1920s, a time characterized by the newly emerging practice of psychotherapy for the treatment of neurosis and when long-term institutional care was the only available solution for psychotic mental illness. By 1940, Erickson had already distinguished himself as someone who had a unique approach to healing. He had published more than 40 papers and would soon come to be known as the world's leading authority on medical hypnosis. Over a period of five decades he illustrated his method of therapy in 119 published case reports. An additional 200 case examples were described in books published by those who studied his approach (O'Hanlon and Hexum, 1990).

Erickson's writings and seminars helped inspire a new generation of therapists. He pioneered strategic and brief approaches to psychotherapy at a time when all psychotherapy was psychoanalytical. His unorthodox practice of bringing members of the family into therapy sessions helped inspire the creation of family therapy. He and a few others ushered in the paradigm shift from the long investigative process that formerly characterized psychotherapy to the realization that effective therapy can and should be brief, internally directed, with a focus on the subject's ability to participate and enjoy life in the present and future. As single-subject research design becomes more common in clinical studies, it is likely that the field will continue to evolve in the direction of individualizing treatment to meet the needs of the patient, a practice that was one of the hallmarks of Erickson's approach.

In addition to his direct contributions, numerous influential figures in the social sciences collaborated with Erickson, including

Gregory Bateson (a scientist and philosopher who contributed to the fields of cybernetics, education, family therapy, and ecology), Margaret Mead (the world-renowned anthropologist who was the first to conduct psychologically oriented field work), Lewis Wolberg (an innovative psychodynamic theorist and pioneer in medical hypnosis), Lawrence Kubie (an eminent psychoanalyst), John Larson (known for his work in the invention of the polygraph), Ernest Rossi, (a leader in the field of mind–body research), and Jay Haley (one of the founders of family therapy).

Family background

Erickson was the offspring of two highly determined individuals. Erickson's father, Albert, lost his father at the age of twelve. Three years later, Albert left Chicago to become a farmer. He had nothing but the clothes on his back and a train ticket. After going as far west as his money would take him, Albert began looking for work in the farming community of Lowell, Wisconsin. He hitched a ride to a farmer's house to seek work as a hired hand. At the house he saw a pretty girl watching him from behind a tree. Albert asked, "Whose girl are you?" She confidently replied, "I'm my daddy's girl." He responded, "Well, you are my girl now." Five years later, Albert and Clara were married. Eventually, they would have nine children and share 73 wedding anniversaries.

Erickson's mother showed a level of determination no less than his father's. When she was sixteen years old, she heard her aunt lamenting on how famous their ancestors were and that no descendent would ever merit the name "Hyland," a much admired relative of the previous generations. Young Clara boldly replied, "When I grow up and get married and have a baby boy, I'm going to name him Hyland!" Milton Hyland Erickson was her second child. He was born in 1901, in a three-sided log cabin with a dirt floor that backed up to a mountain. This was a desolate region of the Nevada Sierras, in a long-since-vanished silver-mining town known as Aurum. As the family grew, Albert and Clara wanted better educational opportunities for the children, so they moved east in a covered wagon.

Childhood

As a child, Erickson was recognized as being different. Although he lived in a rural community with a paucity of printed material, he had an insatiable appetite for reading and amused himself by reading the dictionary for hours at a time. Ironically, he had multiple sensory disorders and apparently had a reading disorder. Erickson later described himself as dyslexic and said that, when he was six, his teacher, Ms Walsh, spent many hours helping him correct his mistranslation of symbols. One such day, Erickson had a sudden burst of insight. His teacher highlighted the most important features of the symbol "3" by turning it on its side. Erickson explains that in a blinding flash of light he suddenly saw the difference between a "3" and an "m." On many other occasions she would use the same method of instruction. She would take something that was very familiar and then suddenly impose it into an area of confusion. Erickson was grateful for what his teacher had taught him and remembered her method, which later became the inspiration for his use of reorientation and a technique known as therapeutic shock.

In addition to problems interpreting symbols, Erickson was colorblind and tone-deaf. Rather than become discouraged by these multiple handicaps, Erickson dedicated himself to careful observation of the world around him. At the age of fifteen, he wrote an article for the magazine *Wisconsin Agriculturists* about the problems of young people living on the farm and why they eventually leave this setting. From his earliest childhood, Erickson was looking for a way to make a difference in the world. This is one reason he had so much admiration for the country doctor who brought hope and comfort into the homes of families who were otherwise frightened and isolated.

Late adolescence

In 1919, Erickson contracted one of the most dreaded diseases of the time, poliomyelitis. His prognosis was poor and he overheard the doctor sadly tell his parents that their boy would be dead by morning. Rather than fall into despair, Erickson reacted with intense anger. He did not feel that anyone had the right to tell a mother that her boy would be dead by morning! In defiance of this morose prediction, Erickson used what little voice he still had to instruct his mother to move his dresser to a certain angle near the foot of his bed. She thought he was delirious but did as he asked. This arrangement allowed Erickson to see down the hallway and out the window of the other room, which faced west. Later, Erickson explained, "I was damned if I would die without seeing one more sunset." After seeing the sunset Erickson lost consciousness for three days.

When Erickson awoke, he could move only his eyes and speak with great difficulty. He was paralyzed in almost every part of his body. All of the independence he had been working to achieve throughout childhood and adolescence suddenly vanished.

Though he was physically trapped by his illness, Erickson still had an unyielding interest in learning. He spent his time as an invalid listening to sounds and interpreting their meaning. For example, he would listen to the sound of footsteps in order to determine who was coming and what sort of mood the person was in. One of his most crucial learning experiences came on a day when Erickson's family left him in the house alone. His body was bound to a rocking chair so that he could have the advantage of sitting up. Erickson did not have much of a view from his position in the room and wished he could be closer to the window so that he could at least have the pleasure of viewing the outside world. As he sat thinking about what it would be like to be closer to the window, he noticed that his rocking chair slowly began to rock. Erickson believed that this was an extraordinary discovery. By merely having the idea of progress he was able to activate some previously unrecognized muscular potential.

During the following weeks and months, Erickson probed his memories for bodily sensations associated with developing movement. He would try to remember what it felt like in his fingers when he held certain objects.

Progress came slowly, in very small portions. First, he got a twitch in one of his fingers. Then he learned to consciously initiate the movement. Then he learned to move more than one finger. Then he learned to move his fingers in uncoordinated ways. Next he developed special resistance exercises that helped him coordinate his movements.

Erickson also studied the movements of his youngest sister, who was just learning to walk. He dissected her behavior into a series of component skills that he could practice for himself. He later explained, "I learned to stand up by watching baby sister learn to stand up: use two hands for a base, uncross your legs, use the knees for a wide base, and then put more pressure on one arm and hand to get up" (Erickson, 1983, p. 13). His willingness to explore the power of ideas and the connection between thinking and the body proved to be key elements in his recovery.

After having a physician at the university recommend vigorous use of his muscles during rehabilitation, Erickson decided he would strengthen his body by paddling a canoe from the Rock River in Milwaukee to the Mississippi and on to St. Louis. He had planned the trip with a companion, but his friend unexpectedly changed his mind at the last minute. Erickson was extraordinarily determined. Because his parents were already uncomfortable with the excursion, he decided not to tell them that he would be handling the canoe and his crutches alone. In the summer of 1922, Erickson was carried to the river by friends. He had two weeks' supply of food, cooking gear, a tent, several textbooks, a few dollars in cash, and a tremendous confidence in his ability to make use of whatever situations he encountered. For instance, when stopped by the first of many dams, Erickson pulled himself up on a pier and waited for someone to pass by and ask why he was there. Erickson found that, when he allowed others to approach him, they were more likely to volunteer help. Along the way he was given temporary jobs by local farmers and fishermen. He earned his board for a 250-mile segment of the trip by cooking for two men who were also traveling the river. On many other occasions he earned his supper by telling stories to fishermen.

The depth of his interest as a student of human behavior deepened during his journey. He was able to see many different ways of living. Six weeks later, Erickson had developed tremendous strength in his arms and shoulders and was able to paddle up against the river current as he headed north from St. Louis back to Milwaukee. He had learned to walk again and was able to carry his canoe on his shoulder. In all, Erickson covered 1,200 river miles and returned home after ten weeks with $5 still in his pocket.

From a state of total paralysis and partial loss of speech, Erickson regained the ability to walk with crutches and speak clearly within eleven months. After approximately two years of rehabilitation, in the fall of 1920, Erickson was able to attend his freshman year at the University of Wisconsin. Erickson's determination to regain the full use of his limbs led him into a journey of discovery beyond what could have initially been hoped.

Professional beginnings

Having participated in research on hypnosis with Clark Hull, Erickson continued to postgraduate medical school in Wisconsin and at the age of 26 qualified for his medical degree and Master of Arts in psychology. He began his career conducting psychological testing and research for the State Board of Control of Wisconsin. Even after earning his medical degree, Erickson would continue to identify himself as both a psychologist and a psychiatrist.

Erickson's first internship in general medicine was at the Colorado General Hospital. He trained in psychiatry at the nearby Colorado Psychopathic Hospital under the direction of Dr Franklin Ebaugh. During his psychiatric residency, Erickson learned to use his disabilities to his advantage. The fact that he was crippled and had to use a cane made him more approachable by his patients. The fact that he did not see the world in the same way as everyone else enabled him to better understand those who had been institutionalized.

With high recommendations from his internship, Erickson was able to secure a position as assistant physician at the highly reputable Rhode Island State Hospital for Mental Diseases. There Erickson conducted intensive studies in the relationship of mental deficiencies to family and environmental factors and published the results. He then advanced to a new appointment at the State Hospital in Worchester, Massachusetts. From 1930 to 1934 he progressed from junior physician to chief research psychiatrist.

Unfortunately, this rapid professional success coincided with the decline of his marriage.

In 1934, Erickson divorced his first wife and was awarded full custody of his three small children. He moved to Michigan, where he became director of psychiatric research and training at Wayne County Hospital, in Eloise, a Detroit suburb. The domestic setback made Erickson even more determined to understand the dynamics of healthy family relationships. A lifelong motto of Erickson's was that mistakes are best embraced as a valuable learning experience.

In 1936, he married Elizabeth Moore, who was a loving mother for her instant family of three children. Over the years, the Erickson family would grow with the birth of five additional children. She and Erickson had a sense of mutual devotion that filled the rest of his lifetime.[1]

Erickson valued family life. His future professional dealings encircled the life of the family. Both at Eloise and throughout thirty years of private practice in Phoenix, the Erickson family lived on site. During the fourteen years at the hospital, the family lived in an apartment in the hospital grounds. During his thirty years of private practice, Erickson's office was in the home, where his children saw him between sessions and interacted with his patients, if his patients wanted that contact. If patients were of an age that Erickson's children might establish friendships with them, Erickson either encouraged the relationship or made it implicitly clear that a friendship was not appropriate.

In his future travels as a lecturer, Erickson was often accompanied by Elizabeth when he traveled. She and other family members, when available, were often used as demonstration subjects.

Erickson's growth was linked to the growth of the family. He was constantly searching for ways to expand his thinking and those around him. At home, he enjoyed presenting a puzzle or a riddle that no one could figure out. There were games, contests, and

---

[1] For more information on Erickson's life with Elizabeth Moore Erickson, see Baker, 2004.

problems presented with great praise for original solutions. This was done in a spirit of fun. It is clear from both his professional legacy and his daily interactions with his family that Erickson truly enjoyed seeking novel and creative solutions to problems. His personal appreciation for the significance of the family translated into pioneering work in the 1940s and 1950s, when Erickson was among the first in the field to use the family to resolve problems and promote individual wellbeing.

In 1947, a minor accident occurred that would eventually alter the direction of Erickson's career. While riding his bicycle, Erickson was knocked to the ground by a dog. The fall resulted in skin lacerations on his arms and forehead. After receiving a tetanus antitoxin, he developed a life-threatening reaction. Due to his severely weakened condition, along with frequent allergy problems and chronic muscle pain, Erickson was no longer able to tolerate the cold and dampness of the Michigan winter. While still in a state of fragile health, Erickson was placed on a train with two medical interns, who accompanied him to Phoenix.

Erickson had been invited to come to the warmer climate by a friend and college, Dr John Larson. At the time, Larson served as superintendent of the Arizona State Hospital. He would soon have Erickson join his staff. Approximately one year after Erickson's move to Phoenix, in the spring of 1949, Larson left his position and moved to California. At that time, Erickson also decided to leave the hospital and transition to private practice work.

Post-polio syndrome

In 1953, Erickson became severely ill with what is now recognized as post-polio syndrome. During this time his pain was extraordinary. He experienced muscle cramps so severe that some muscles literally tore themselves apart. Even during these moments of great hardship and confinement to bed, he found the energy and concentration necessary to accept phone calls from individuals seeking his aid. His genuine concern for others provided a welcome distraction from his own physical pain.

After recovering from what was believed at the time to be a second attack of polio, Erickson had lost many of the muscles in his arm, back, abdomen, and legs. However, he still managed to maintain a busy lecture schedule, including travel across the country and aboard. Though not as severe as the 1953 attack, Erickson endured further episodes of intense pain and confinement to bed.

The 1950s would be one of the most eventful periods of Erickson's career. It was at this time that he became a nationally known figure. He was featured in popular news media such as *Life* magazine. He was also consulted as an expert in psychology and human behavior by famous athletes, the US military, the FBI, and the Aerospace Laboratory of Medicine. In 1957, Erickson co-founded the American Society of Clinical Hypnosis (ASCH). Earlier he and four colleagues formed Seminars on Hypnosis which taught medical, dental, and psychological uses of hypnosis throughout the country. He and his colleagues agreed to use $50,000 from that enterprise to fund the educational arm of ASCH. Erickson served as founding president of ASCH for two years and as founding editor of the ASCH journal for ten years.

By 1967, the continued deterioration of muscles forced Erickson to use a wheelchair during his travels. While in Delaware, September 1967, speaking at what was to be one of his final lectures on the road; Erickson remarked that he was learning to find joy in all of the new things he could experience from the vantage point of a wheelchair. By 1969, traveling became too exhausting, so Erickson focused his energy on his activities at his home office, which included writing papers, editing, seeing patients and training therapists. Using the skills that as a youth enabled him to survive polio, Erickson refused to live life as an invalid and, much like the archetypal "wounded healer," he found the inner resources necessary to continue helping others for as long as possible.

His compelling contributions did not go unnoticed. In 1976, at the Seventh Congress of the International Society of Hypnosis, Erickson became the first recipient of the Benjamin Franklin Gold Medal award for the highest achievement in the theory and practice of hypnotism.

The later years

Despite a lifetime of chronic pain and illness, Erickson embraced a love of the life he had been given. Through his suffering, Erickson learned to value humor and the simple pleasures of life. For instance, having become infirm, he attached a horn to his wheel-chair and joked with some of his patients about being an "old codger." During the teaching seminars conducted from his office, nearly all of the exercises were approached in a humorous manner that brought a sense of playful enjoyment to the learning process (Zeig, 1980).

While training therapists, Erickson taught one of his favorite lessons using what looked like a large granite rock. He kept this prop by him in his office and at the right moment would reach down and begin the arduous task of lifting it to his lap. Watching this was difficult for the students. They had to struggle with whether or not they should risk insulting Erickson by offering assistance or just sit and watch a frail old man struggle to lift a granite rock into his lap. When it was finally resting in his lap, Erickson would look around at each of the students and then slowly lift it again and, without warning, lunge it effortlessly through the air into the lap of a stunned student. What appeared to be a heavy rock was actually an almost weightless piece of foam. Erickson would fix his eyes on the student and say, "Not everything is as it seems!" The shock would soon wear off but the lesson would never be forgotten.

Erickson's greatest pleasure seemed to be derived from community building. Over the years there were literally hundreds of patients, and students who were also receiving therapy, who developed valued and long-lasting relationships with Erickson family members. Twenty-five years after Erickson's death, many of those friendships still flourish. This flexibility and creative use of resources added elements of sharing, learning together, social support, and extended family to Erickson's therapy.

As he aged, Erickson's physical complications multiplied exponentially. In 1974, he commented to Rossi that the pain had become so intense and pervasive that he felt like a stranger in his own body. Toward the end of his life he had great difficulty lifting his right arm and he had very little strength in his hands. Many of the muscles in his face and mouth were paralyzed. Despite these physical obstacles, Erickson continued to use what strength he had left to provide therapy and training to individuals from around the world.

At the time of his death, Tuesday evening, March 25, 1980, Erickson's teaching schedule was already filled through the end of the year and there were unconfirmed applications that would have extended his appointments far into the following year. Erickson remained productive up until the very last moments of his life, playing his part to make a difference in the world.

As can be seen in this brief biographical sketch, Erickson's life was characterized by determination, resiliency, and hope. The ideas that he advocated within his therapy are the same ideas exemplified by how he lived his life. He had a profound appreciation for the strength that comes from a willingness to establish meaningful objectives and then doing something in relation to that goal. For Erickson, progress was not dependent on things going "his way." He derived intrinsic satisfaction by acquiring some new understanding. By seeking to learn something from his physical disabilities, Erickson understood how to provide hope to those who no longer felt they could help themselves. He fostered resiliency in his patients through the strategic activation of latent abilities. This was an important part of his philosophy of healing. He believed that all people have within them the answer to whatever challenges they face.

As will be seen in the following pages, Erickson knew how to accomplish the "impossible" by finding some small thing that can be done. Building on a framework of small successes, he reinforced resiliency within the individual by engaging immediate successes that reach into the future.

Milton H. Erickson will continue to be remembered for his determination, patient perseverance, humanity, and unending love of learning. From these he benefited personally while at the same time creating a broader spectrum for the field of psychotherapy and benefiting people around the world, decades after his death.

Part I

Foundations of Healing and Health

Chapter 1

Introduction

What is more important, technique or understanding? If after reading this book the reader is mostly excited about the new techniques that have been discovered, then the book should be read again in order to arrive at the main point.

Most will agree that there is a difference in status between a technician and an expert. A technician is paid less money, has less education, and is assigned to tasks that can be described using step-by-step procedures found in a technical manual. In contrast, an expert is someone who applies reason to problem-solving endeavors and when necessary creates new techniques to address novel circumstances. When considering the diversity and complexity of human problems, it is difficult to imagine how someone functioning at the technician level could make appreciable gains. It is a matter of common sense to recognize that a therapist-technician, a person entirely dependent upon treatment manuals and step-by-step procedures, is not as well prepared to meet the unique needs of each individual patient as the therapist-expert, a person who exercises reason and discovery within the context of a helping relationship.

Expert therapy requires clinical judgment. Clinical judgment is in many ways dependent on the practitioner's understanding of healing and mental health. Some of this understanding develops over time through experience and exposure. However, the educated professional benefits from having an intellectually informed starting point. Such a start does not come from memorizing excessive jargon or becoming lost in an obscure analysis of minutiae. Instead, it grows forth from an appreciation for the fundamental dynamics of health and healing. So that is where this book begins.

Although it is possible to employ powerful psychotherapeutic techniques without knowledge of the broader understanding from which they were derived, success under these circumstances is more likely to depend on random chance rather than skillful discernment. In order to appreciate fully the clinical strategies described in this book, it is important, first, to develop a conceptual understanding of how mental healing occurs.

Although the following principles may seem academic, they serve the practical purpose of providing the logic behind clinical judgment. In order to individualize treatment in the way that Erickson did, it is necessary to understand the foundational principles that facilitate commonsense reasoning. Therapists who tailor their treatment to the needs of the patient, using an integrated model of therapy, require some means of determining the proper problem-solving principles to apply to each individual case.

When equipped with an underlying philosophy of healing and growth, the practitioner is able to recognize a wide array of therapeutic options and determine which direction is best given a certain set of circumstances. In contrast, to study therapeutic techniques without the benefit of an appropriate philosophical base makes no more sense than a lifeguard learning how to swim but without recognizing how to find the shore. In the following pages, the reader will be exposed to a parsimonious explanation of core objectives. Using a minimum number of theoretical constructs, the text offers a foundational understanding that will act as a guide for navigating occasionally bewildering clinical circumstances.

Once a person knows where to go, the next step is to know how to get there. In the second part of the book, the focus shifts to the intellectual tools used in skillful therapy. Because these tools are used with intention and toward a specific end, they are most appropriately identified as "strategies."

This book examines core strategies that were woven through and through Erickson's work. Each strategic principle is then broken down into several techniques that share a common function. To help bring to life these clinical strategies and to provide the experience of witnessing masterful clinical work, this book contains numerous clinical examples from Erickson and others. Those who have systematically studied Erickson's work will notice that many of these case examples have never before been published. In order to make clearer the core function of any given technique, the overarching concepts have been paired with simple analogies, folk wisdom, and illustrations from other schools of psychotherapy. The reader should not become distracted over which school of thought the book is describing but instead seek to recognize the timelessness and universal nature of these strategic principles. This scaffold framework not only helps the reader better understand the interventions and strategies employed by Erickson, but, more importantly, points beyond the finite limits of Erickson's achievements to an ever-expanding tradition of exploratory and innovative work by which he was characterized.

Erickson approached his patients with the type of admiration and respect that comes from an appreciation for the complexity and uniqueness of human life. His therapy was not based on a rigid application of step-by-step procedures. Because flexibility is an important hallmark of Erickson's approach to healing, it is *clinical understanding* rather than rigid rules that *must drive the decision-making process*. While reading this book, there is no need to memorize what was said or done by Erickson in response to a particular situation. Rather, the reader will hopefully finish the book feeling better prepared to spontaneously develop novel solutions to complex and diverse clinical circumstances. This is an exploratory humanistic endeavor that helps balance scientific reductionism. As it was with Erickson, the thinking practitioner must be willing to experiment and be prepared to develop new therapeutic approaches for each client.

Through an extensive consideration of his written works, decades of lectures, hundreds of case examples, and his day-to-day behavior at home, the authors have attempted to resurrect Erickson's voice. The idea that several different techniques can serve the same function and the belief that every intervention should be carried out with careful intention come directly from the teaching of Milton Erickson. After reading Part I of the book, the reader will be able to recognize fundamental dynamics of healing and of the clinical relationship. This philosophical model will then serve as a context for the selection and implementation of clinical strategies. Part II will then provide a description of each strategy. These are introduced in a broad and simplistic manner, followed by a more elaborate and complex examination of the clinical techniques derived from a given strategy. While studying these techniques, it is important to recognize that it is the broad concepts, and not the specific techniques, that are used to facilitate the development of an unlimited number of unique solutions. Although this text is not meant to serve as a summation of the clinical work of Milton Erickson, it does provide a solid basis for recognizing how he learned to approach health-related problem-solving endeavors.

Chapter 2

The Human Condition

This chapter examines the unstated expectations people hold and the insidious problem of perfectionism. A case example as told by Erickson during one of his many seminars has been selected so that the reader can contrast his or her initial conclusions about Erickson's work with the book's analysis. The case report in this chapter will be elaborated on in further detail in Chapter 8. The narrative has been divided in this way to help illustrate the multi-dimensional nature of Erickson's work. It is important to recognize that there is not just one point to be gleaned from each case example. As intended by Erickson, each story is a metaphor designed to communicate timeless lessons that are difficult to bind up in an explicit construct or theory.

Case report: The man who cursed life

> A man was brought to Erickson in a wheelchair, with arms and knees fixed to the chair. He was angry and cursed the fact that he had spent the last eleven years paralyzed by painful arthritis. He could move only his head and had some slight movement in one thumb. He was completely dependent on his wife, who dressed him, put him in his wheelchair every morning, then fed him, and put him to bed at night. All the while, he continued cursing about his unhappy life.
>
> Erickson's statements were simple and to the point. He reproached the man for his lack of movement: "You have a thumb that will move and you better move it! You better exercise your _____, _____ thumb every day in order to pass the _____ time." [Blank spaces indicate use of expletives.]
>
> The man responded to Erickson's medical advice by becoming defiant, wanting to prove to Erickson that he could, "wiggle the damn thumb all day and all night, and all week, and all month,"," and it would, "not do a damn bit of good!"

The man went home absolutely determined to make his point. But, as he continued to exercise his thumb, he suddenly noticed movement in his index finger, the digit most likely to be affected by movement of the thumb. As the exercising progressed he became able to move more fingers. He became fascinated by this. Each new sign of progress kept him absorbed in finding out how many more little movements he could get out of his fingers. Then he became able to move his wrist, and then finally his arms.

These exercises became the man's method of passing time. Then, a year after his first appointment, Erickson gave him the task of painting a small cabin. The man responded by swearing as he informed Erickson that if he had any common sense he would not send a man with such limited movement to paint a cabin. Erickson persisted.

The assignment took him about three weeks. By the end of the summer he increased his speed and was able to paint a stucco duplex in a week's time. Following these accomplishments, he got a job as a truck driver. Next he decided he should join a fraternal order and was soon elected president of that order. During his ongoing work with Erickson, the man decided he needed a college education and went to college.

Some symptoms of the man's severe arthritis remained. Despite this condition Erickson explains, "He looks forward to the rainy season each year and the three to seven days during which he will be confined to bed with painful arthritis." The man was able to tolerate the intermittent bedridden condition because it gave him an opportunity to catch up on good books he wanted to read. Rather than being viewed as a relapse, the residual arthritis was identified as producing a "vacation."

(Erickson, 1957)

Because of the seemingly incredible nature of this case report and most others described in this book, it is very important to pay close attention to what was actually achieved and what was not. It is a mistake to be seduced by the idea that Erickson's use of hypnosis produced some sort of magical cure. Wonderful as the outcome was for the man with arthritis, it is essential to recognize that he was *not* cured of arthritis. On the contrary, there remained certain circumscribed moments in which his problem was just as intense as when he first came for therapy. The residual arthritis was so debilitating that he was again temporarily confined to bed. However, the therapy was highly successful in that he was no longer an invalid.

The first major point to recognize is that perfection is not an appropriate therapeutic goal. Although he was often admired for his powers of persuasion, Erickson was careful to avoid misplaced notions of control. He did not try to make people conform to a standard of perfection. In Erickson's words, "perfection is not a human attribute" (1973/2001b, p. 14). Accordingly, he warned of the complications of striving for a *total* cure. Instead, Erickson remained focused on the task of promoting the patient's health, as imperfect as it may be. He felt it important to search for some small good that could be accomplished in relation to the patient's current situation.

Erickson approached therapy with the premise that all suffering can be reduced. Although pain in life is unavoidable, it does not have to be overwhelming. Painful events can instead be perceived as an inconvenience, a problem, a challenge, something where there can be some sort of improvement (Erickson-Klein, 1990, p. 273).[1]

As will often occur, one small gain can lead to other unexpected outcomes and even cascade into completely unanticipated benefits. As with the case of the man with arthritis, Erickson admitted that he initially had no idea the patient would make such remarkable progress. The man had been putting most of his energy into making the problem worse. Once that energy was shifted toward identifying unrecognized possibilities, seemingly impossible circumstances were transcended. If Erickson had attempted to cure the man, he would most certainly have failed. Instead he hoped that some amount of good could be accomplished.

---

[1] Because somatic pain is a warning signal that something is wrong with the body, the psychological treatment of pain is appropriate once the causal factors are known and medical treatment is under way.

The second major point is that living requires effort. This is often over-looked in a culture of modern conveniences. In addition to being imperfect, people need to work hard in order to function well. Healthy muscles require constant exercise. Healthy brains require ongoing stimulation and effortful processing. Healthy families require constant attention and involvement. In most of his clinical work, Erickson rarely used words or phrases that implied a passive role for the patient. He found stimulating ways of encouraging patients to be actively engaged in their own healing processes. Having grown up on a farm, he fully appreciated the meaning of, "You must do your share of the work." He understood the feeling of satisfaction that comes after a hard day's toil.

Accordingly, Erickson put a great deal of time and energy into each clinical case. He kept meticulous notes, writing down everything that was said during a session. Then he planned and reviewed every word and action that might occur in following sessions and what impact it might have. In some cases, he drove to patients' houses in order to better understand the setting from which they came. What this meant was that Erickson often spent more time preparing for a session than in the sessions themselves. Erickson's opinion was that the results of each problem-solving endeavor will be proportional to the amount of effort invested in finding a solution (Hughes and Rothovius, 1996, p. 236).

In the case of the man with arthritis, Erickson put him to work first exercising his thumb. This eventually progressed into painting houses. Engaging the patient in productive effort, as small as it initially was, eventually produced a profound effect. Similarly, Erickson taught other patients with severely debilitating pain to take advantage of moments when they are feeling better in order to be productive (Erickson-Klein, 1990).

Regardless of the disability or state of health, a lack of effort results in lack of progress. Perhaps this is why many clinicians wisely avoid enabling passivity by adhering to the maxim, "Never work harder than the patient." As Erickson (1952/2001b) explains, "Whatever the part played by the hypnotist may be, the role of the subjects involve [*sic*] the greater amount of active functioning—functioning which derives from the capabilities, learnings, and experiential history of their total personalities" (p. 27). Because the active involvement of the patient is so important, the clinician should avoid fixating on what the patient must *stop* doing. Growth-oriented therapy focuses on what the patient can start doing.

Next, it is important to recognize that life involves a process of *reciprocal determinism*. The world of human ideas and experiential reality is impacted by the physical universe. At the same time, human thinking provides impetus for the events of the external world. Erickson alluded to this dynamic while referring to the centuries-old philosophy, "As a man thinketh, so he is" (Erickson and Rossi, 1979, p. 262). In the case above, the man was given a new perspective on arthritis. Erickson explains, "Although he still limps a little, he has a nice healthy attitude." In other words, the man learned to think better of his situation and adapt to his physical limitations.

Erickson used this case to illustrate the importance of accepting and finding use for the patient's disability. This is the essence of adaptation and resiliency. It can be said in very general terms that where adaptation and resiliency end, death begins.

In order not to be immobilized by life's challenges, a person must have the capacity to accept undesirable circumstances. This idea was communicated well by Tyler Hamilton, a cycling contestant in the 2003 Tour de France. During the first stage of the race, he was in a crash that fractured his collarbone. Despite intense pain he managed to complete the race and take fourth place. When asked how he was able to accomplish this remarkable feat, Hamilton said that he learned to accept the pain. Once he stopped struggling against it he was able to make the necessary adjustments in posture, balance, and thinking. This is perhaps what Erickson meant when he described rigid inflexibility as the most general problem to be dealt with in psychotherapy (Zeig, 1980).

Flexibility and adaptation are as essential to resiliency as acceptance is to learning. If a person continues to struggle and fight intractable changes to the environment, mind, or body, energy is wasted and recovery is hindered. For instance, Betty Alice Erickson recalls the case of a five-year-old boy who was traumatized after witnessing a terrible automobile accident. The little boy had seen a man lying on the street with a severed leg. It left a disturbing image in his mind. He talked about it a great deal and drew pictures of the leg and the body. The unfortunate scene seemed to be ever present in his mind. The boy's parents tried talking to him, explaining that automobile accidents were rare, and asked him to forget about it and no longer draw pictures of it. But the youngster remained fixated on the horrible sight.

Betty Alice Erickson sought consultation so she could better understand the essential dynamics. Erickson told her that the little boy was faced with the possibility of his own parents suffering this catastrophe and, as little children do, was worried about his own future. These were feelings he would not be able to understand. Erickson indicated that dealing with these types of worries on a logical basis never works. He advised that the parents should take one of the pictures of the man with the severed leg, and admire it. They should let the boy know how well he had captured the sight of the blood. They should ask about details in the picture, such as, "Was that the right distance to have between the man and his severed leg?" The expression on the man's face should be examined with the child—and the boy praised for his accuracy in that as well. Then the child should be asked very seriously to draw a picture of the man *after* the doctors had helped him.

"That little boy," Erickson explained, "is looking for a way out of his impossible dilemma." Doctors, at his age, were still categorized as supreme authorities who could do wonderful and amazing things. As Erickson predicted, drawing a picture of the man, *after* the doctors had helped, gave the child a sense of closure and the type of hope needed to live happily.

If human thought is closely linked to emerging realities, then it is only logical that the most important point to *communicate in therapy is the idea that change is possible.* That is why Erickson avoided promising cures that seemed impossible and sometimes paradoxically asserted the inevitability of failure. As he explains,

> You start building up in the patient a philosophy that allows him to accept some degree of failure. You suggest to your impotent patient that you regret exceedingly that no matter how well you succeed with him, you're going to fail ten percent of the time. And

you express that intense regret that he's going to fail ten percent of the time and you regret it. But what you're really telling him is that he's going to succeed ninety percent of the time.

(Erickson, 1962a)

Erickson often used this approach with a patient who was absolutely convinced he would fail. He phrased his statements in such a way that change suddenly seemed possible while still leaving some space for the acceptance of imperfection.

Erickson would sometimes end a trance by stating, "All good things must come to an end." This is one of the most profound dilemmas encountered by living creatures. Our reality is bound to a frail body that will eventually expire. As a person who had been crippled by polio, Erickson not only understood but also was a model of acceptance of human frailty. His response to this human condition is reminiscent of the biblical saying, "Your body is a temple." *Erickson's therapy was one that always pointed to the goodness and importance of the body.* As Erickson recognized early in his career, "One need only call to mind a small boy proudly displaying his muscles to realize how important a sense of pride, trust and confidence in one's own body is for a normal healthy outlook upon life" (Erickson, 1941/2001a, p. 4). In this way, he *defined the individual as the unit of change in psychotherapy* and a positive clinical outcome as, "the opportunity of directing every intensity of the personality into making use of the body. This serves the purpose of helping you bring about therapeutic results" (Erickson, 1957). The implicit element of this philosophy is the social context in which the change occurs.

Although the individual may be the unit of change, it is often the *helping relationship* that ignites the transformation process, resulting in greater hope and increased resiliency. Such help may come from one person, such as a parent, therapist, or good friend. Or there may be a group of individuals invested in helping one another, such as in group therapy, family therapy, or community support groups. Each of these has its own unique benefits.

While explaining the transformation of the man with arthritis, Erickson simply commented that he knew the man could move his thumb and that the thumb was connected to other bones in the body, which were in turn connected to other bones, and so on. In other words, as long as there is life and movement, some part of the body can always be brought into play against the disability. But this activation of internal resources will not occur as long as the latent potential remains unrecognized.

Unfortunately, it is not uncommon for those in distress to isolate their efforts to the activation of the part of the body formally assigned a specific task. If that effort is not successful, then eventually the person decides that the situation really is hopeless and thus surrenders to disability. However, from his own experiences with polio, Erickson recognized that other parts of the mind and body can compensate for even a substantial loss of ability.

Before coming to therapy the man could not move his index finger through a conscious activation of those muscles. However, while wiggling his thumb he was able to produce movement in the finger attached to it. This discovery highlighted, in microcosm, the compensatory method of using muscles that had some strength to produce movement in muscles that had atrophied. Under Erickson's guidance, the man took all of the energy that had been wasted on profanity and put it into exercising his thumb, fingers, and arms, and then into full body movement. In this way, the progress was cumulative. He discovered that his situation truly was not as impossible as he had once believed. This case report illustrates that there was no "magic" in Erickson's work. Instead, it was the activation of hope and resiliency that resulted in a beneficial clinical outcome.

Chapter 3

Mental Health and Healing

This chapter examines in a holistic manner the process of healing and its interface with mental-health care. The concept of healing is examined in relation to the pursuit of mental health. Although some have argued that the concept of mental illness unnecessarily pathologizes those who have encountered difficult circumstances (Duncan, Miller, and Sparks, 2004), in this book the term "mental health" refers to a personal victory in the challenge to survive and thrive. "Healing" is used to refer to the extraordinary capacity of the mind and body to recover from injury. Accordingly, the chapter begins with a case example that nicely illustrates Erickson's faith in the resiliency of his patients.

Case report: Rebecca

A seven-year-old girl named Rebecca was brought to Erickson's office fully wrapped in a protective blanket. She had not been able to leave her house for several weeks. The thought of going outside was incredibly painful for her and brought on violent symptoms such as vomiting, diarrhea, incontinence, tachycardia, and fainting. Erickson began therapy by discussing in a slow and systematic manner just how much she thought he should unwrap and how much of the blanket should remain in place. This was a long and slow process intended to build a sense of trust and safety. Then, just as carefully, he reviewed with her just how much she felt that she should tell him.

Her story goes like this. As she was coming home from school, a large dog, a German Shepherd, had bitten her. This frightened her horribly. Then the owners of the dog came out and harshly scolded her for bothering their dog. Later they made it clear that they resented having to pay to have their dog sent for observation. After recovering from the dog bite, Rebecca was walking home from school and again was attacked by the dog. The owners had decided not to lock up the dog because they felt it was entitled to exercise. Again, the owners rebuked the little girl, telling her that they were going to take legal action against her parents. Rebecca stayed home all weekend recovering from the second dog bite. On Monday, she started out for school but got only as far as the sidewalk and returned home not feeling well. The next day she got only as far as the front porch before becoming ill. The third day she would not leave the house.

Erickson's first response was to justify her fear and the associated symptoms. With a look of astonishment he told her, "I am surprised that you are such a strong and healthy girl!" Referring to the traumatic events, he explained, "I am surprised that you are not a lot worse. I am surprised that your heart does not beat faster. I am surprised that you are so strong and healthy and that your fainting does not last longer and that you do not have more diarrhea!" Later, Erickson explained his approach by saying, "I had to give that girl some good opinion of her body and her behavior." After sitting and listening to Erickson praise her strengths, Rebecca began to develop a different opinion of herself. She began laughing and joking and wanted to see Erickson's dog, which he had described as a harmless basset. After six more visits, Rebecca required no further therapy.

(Erickson, 1961a)

After suffering a terrible trauma, such as the one described above, how does healing occur? What is it that makes a person return to a state in which he or she is ready to deal with the external world? Erickson's psychotherapeutics consisted of a constellation of procedures used for the purpose of communicating the idea that "you have the capacity for healing and health." In the case of Rebecca, Erickson directly and convincingly communicated the idea that she was a strong and healthy girl. He reaffirmed the goodness of her body. He helped her feel courageous. Having accepted these ideas, she was able to heal and thereby return to a state of mental health.

Healing is the activation of inner resources during the process of recovery. As will be seen in Chapter 9, a great deal of healing comes from emphasizing positive attributes located in the individual and then building on them incrementally. This is why Erickson argued throughout his career that cures are not the product of suggestion but instead result from the reassociation of experience (Lankton, 1997/2003). Erickson's emphasis on identifying and thereby encouraging a positive view of the goodness of the body is illustrated well in the case of Rebecca.

In general, it can be said that health is an active process that originates internally. We are all familiar with the doctor's advice to eat well and get lots of exercise. But health is much more than the decision to feed oneself and vigorously move about. There needs to be a willingness to build up one's self in all regards. Health is the pursuit of meaningful labor, a vigilant readiness to avoid harm and live a long life, or the creation of a happy home. These are the long-term goals that provide a sense of direction and meaning. Then there are the innumerable daily acts of health such as taking a deep breath, talking with a good friend, caring for a garden, or setting aside time for a moment of solitude. These short-term goals provide motivation to remain engaged in an ever-changing environment. With these come the recognition and acceptance of one's limitations and human fragility. All of these objectives come from a willingness to engage various capacities of the mind and body.

Whenever possible, health should be guarded rather than having to be restored. Erickson's approach to mental health was proactive whenever possible. For instance, in the 1960s Betty Alice Erickson and her husband David Elliott adopted a Vietnamese baby to join their two young sons. Betty Alice is blue-eyed with fair skin and David and the two little boys were also blond and blue-eyed. During this time period, interracial adoptions were quite uncommon and even illegal in many states.

Kimberly's obvious differences were likely to cause her great discomfort at home and at school. Erickson, however, made the little girl's dark skin, dark hair, and eyes a wonderful distinction. She became his "Gingerbread Girl." He affectionately used the nickname and wrote special cards and letters to his Gingerbread Girl. When the family visited, he always had gingerbread cookies on his table that only his Gingerbread Girl could hand out—much to her brothers' annoyance. He even had a gingerbread girl doll made for her by her Aunt Roxanna.

Erickson and Kimberly had many special conversations about gingerbread. "Gingerbread," Kimberly proudly announced to her brothers, "is brown and sweet and a very special treat that people don't have all the time." She told them proudly, "Me and Grandpa talk about it a lot."

When Kimberly became a US citizen, Erickson sent her a hand-drawn card that said, "Congratulations! The Gingerbread Girl is now an American Gingerbread Girl!"

It is not possible to know how Kimberly would have otherwise handled her physiological differences from the rest of her family. But Erickson, as a person outside her nuclear family, defined her dark skin as exceptional in very special, sweet, and spicy "gingerbread" ways. Even the envy of her brothers added to the positive status of her differences.

When Kimberly started school, her Kindergarten teacher was Hispanic. As Kimberly was being driven home from her first day, she turned to her mother and stated with pride, "I have a gingerbread lady for a teacher. I showed her my arm and told her I was a gingerbread girl too."

Rather than objectify health as a clinical endpoint, we should see it as a lifelong process. Kimberly's comment reflected a healthy development in her personality. In the same way that health is an ongoing effort, so is healing. Because the outside world contains a constant series of biological and psychological threats the need for healing is constant. Or as Erickson would say, *"life is a continuous process of rehabilitation"* (Rossi, 2004, p.9). Every day brings a new opportunity to work cheerfully with one's limitations, without complaint or regret (*ibid.*). Lasting health requires more than successful treatment.

A general reference that Erickson would make was his observation of psychotic patients who have stopped eating or anorexic patients who were hospitalized and treated by being tube-fed several thousand calories a day. Yet, even with this abundant caloric intake, malnutrition remained a life-threatening problem. The tube feeding was an example of treatment without the activation of healing.

A similar observation was made by Viktor Frankl (1973). He cites the case of a patient cured of gangrene by having his leg amputated; then, finding himself unable to cope with the loss of his limb, he committed suicide. Thus healing is something separate from treatment. Treatments are interventions coming from the outside. Healing is something that occurs from within and involves all of the body's systems. A similar distinction was articulated by a nineteenth-century physician who stated, "I dressed the wound but it was God who healed it." The essential point to be understood is that, whether biological or psychological, it is the capacities and resources of the patient that produce sustainable health.

The most significant distinction between treatment and healing is that treatment cannot operate independently of healing. Healing is a product of the collective resources of the body. In contrast, a treatment is an external influence enacted in an effort to direct the individual toward a state of health. Similarly, the definition of a drug is, "an *exogenous* chemical not necessary for normal cellular functioning that significantly alters the functions of certain cells of the body when taken in relatively low doses" (Carlson, 2004, p. 101). A drug becomes medicinal when it directs the functions of certain cells toward a sustainable state of health. A psychological treatment is also an exogenous agent, "produced from without;" however, its substance is behavioral rather than chemical. Whether medical or psychological, treatment and healing have a cumulative effect but treatment cannot succeed without a simultaneous process of healing.

Therefore, the question the clinician must consider for each patient is, "What does this person need in order to experience the innate capacity to heal?" To promote this process effectively, one must, "Let patients know that they *are* going to be cured and that it will take place *within* them" (Erickson, 1965b). In some cases, the idea may be communicated in a single statement. But, with more severely damaged patients, progress toward mental health requires a long slow process of discovering a new reality orientation.

Reality orientation comes from a combination of learning, memory, and immediate sensory experience. Biologically, these exist in separate anatomical locations that are connected through a complex roadway of neural networks. Life experiences literally become physical territory within the brain, places that can be journeyed to or away from. The movement of conscious awareness to and from these regions is initiated either internally by a train of thought or by external cues, a recognition that a piece of that reality experience still exists in the external world. From a functional perspective, *mental health increases in proportion to the individual's ability to journey without inhibition to the different regions of the mind in which life experiences are stored.* Without such ability, the individual is less effective in recognizing and dealing with the external world. The resulting difficulties are then classified as "symptoms," which may be manifest in numerous realms ranging from cognitive functions and affect to physiology and general health. The important point to recognize is that mental health is not something that can be standardized and then forced upon a patient. It is a subjective victory that is uniquely defined by each person's background of life experiences and learnings. The Ericksonian perspective on mental health requires a unique therapeutic relationship, one in which the practitioner is able to work within the patient's frames of reference in order to achieve an outcome that is meaningful to the patient.

Chapter 4

The Role of the Clinician

This chapter describes the type of relationship used by Erickson to elicit change in his patients. The chapter begins with a case example that illustrates how Erickson would function as an expert but without acting superior. This case is a particularly telling example because it is an adult speaking to a child. Yet, as the adult, Erickson continues to respect the child's right to personal choice. The case report in this chapter will be elaborated on in further detail again in Chapter 11. While at this point we are mostly interested in the nature of the therapeutic relationship, the second glimpse at this case will provide an important insight into the therapeutic strategy Erickson employed.

Case report: Johnny's big chassis

A father and mother brought their twelve-year-old son to Erickson, stating, "This boy has wet his bed every night of the week since he was an infant!" They explained that they had reached the absolute limit of their patience. They had attempted what they considered to be every known method of curing him. His father had whipped him, made him clean his sheets, made him go without food and water and even tried rubbing Johnny's face in the urine soaked sheets. The parents had attempted every kind of punishment imaginable, but the boy continued wetting the bed. Erickson responded to their dictatorial comments with an equally strong authoritarian statement, "Now he is my patient. I don't want you interfering with any therapy that I do on your son." Then he sized up the situation, "You want a dry bed. I'll do the therapy and you let me and your son alone. You let me make all of my arrangements with your son and keep your mouths shut and be courteous to my patient." In their desperation, the parents agreed to his terms.

In a private meeting with twelve-year-old Johnny, Erickson described how he had given his instructions to the parents. Johnny was pleased with the conditions that had been established. Next Erickson told Johnny, "You know, your father is six foot two inches. He is a great big, powerful, husky man. You are only a twelve-year-old kid. How tall are you?" Johnny replied he was five foot nine inches. Next Erickson asked, "What does your father weigh?" "Two hundred twenty pounds." Erickson noted that the father was a full 220 pounds and not the least bit fat.

Next, Johnny was asked how much he weighed. Erickson acted astonished at the answer, "You weigh 170 pounds and you are a twelve-year-old kid, aren't you? Do you suppose that it has taken a lot of body energy and body strength to build that great big, beautiful chassis on a twelve-year old kid?"

Looking him over, Erickson added, "Think of all the muscle you have got and the strength that you have got. You have been putting an awful lot of energy into building all of that in twelve short years. What do you think you will be when you are as old as your father? Just a shrimpy six foot two inches, weighing only 220 pounds? Or do you think you will be taller than your father and heavier than your father? You are just twelve years old and you already weigh 170. Your great big father only weighs 50 pounds more than you. And he is a lot older than you!"

Johnny pondered these questions obviously pleased with this new and different perspective. He had never considered his physical growth as a significant accomplishment.

Erickson continued, "Now they have told me to cure you of wetting the bed. And they have told me of all of their misbehavior in trying to do it. Well, now, let's get it straight, Johnny. I'm not going to cure you of wetting the bed. Instead I am going to tell you a few things. You have spent an awful lot of energy and strength on building this great big beautiful chassis on a twelve-year-old boy. You are going to be a football star in college. You are going to be an athlete in college. You haven't got far to go! Only a lousy 51 pounds to outweigh your father! And you have got nine years until you are an adult, nine years to gain 51 pounds! You can do that. You know it and I know it."

(Erickson, 1964a)

22

In psychotherapy, *the clinician's principal role is to act as a catalyst, using the mind and body together as the primary remedial force*. In this role the practitioner is responsible for helping the patient recognize new possibilities. In the preceding example, a boy who can see no alternative to a lifetime of bedwetting is stimulated with novel ideas that create a resilient hope for future possibilities. As Erickson explained, "You could see Johnny's mind turning handsprings in all directions. He was getting a new body image of himself as a man" (Erickson, 1964a).

Early in his career, Erickson recognized that psychotherapy is a *learning process*. He argued that the role of the clinician is to help facilitate the re-education of the patient (Erickson, 1948/2001, p. 4). This objective is accomplished through a process of experiential learning that is best facilitated through active therapies such as hypnotherapy, Gestalt therapy, psychodrama, etc. While describing his creative use of hypnotherapy, Erickson explained, "Effective results … derive only from the patient's activities. *The therapist merely stimulates the patient into activity* [our emphasis]" (p. 3). Similarly, research has shown that when attitudes are formed as a result of direct personal experience they predict behavior better then when they are formed as a result of exposure to secondhand information (Fazio and Zanna, 1981).

As a catalyst, the therapist must use clinical judgment in order to determine how to guide the patient in the learning process. The patient's task is to work toward a new understanding of his experiential life. In contrast to the type of education that occurs in an academic setting, in psychotherapy it is not the ideas or opinions of the therapist that are important. As stated by Erickson (1948/2001), "Such re-education is, of course, necessarily in terms of the patient's life experiences, his understandings, memories, attitudes, and ideas" (p. 3). In this type of therapy, the therapist's role is active rather than passive, creating the impetus for change by guiding the patient through a process of growth and discovery (Lankton, 2001/2003, p. 7).

While journeying along side the patient, through various experiential realities, it is vitally important for the clinician to recognize the importance of eliciting the cooperation and participation of the patient. Erickson defined this dynamic in a 1966 lecture, stating,

"In the relationship between patient and clinician, you have one goal in common. The patient wants some type of care and you are prepared to give the desired care. There are two people joined together, working for a common goal—the welfare of the patient." However, this type of cooperative relationship cannot be established by following rigid procedures and fixed methods of therapy. "The complexity of human behavior and its underlying motivations make necessary a cognizance of the multitude of factors existing in any situation arising between two personalities engaged in a joint activity" (Erickson, 1952/2001b, p. 27). In other words, the clinician should be ready to cooperate with the needs of the patient to better facilitate reciprocal cooperation.

Erickson believed strongly in the utility of reciprocal interactions (Erickson-Elliott, and Erickson-Klein, 1991). Therefore the therapeutic relationship should be characterized by comradeship and reciprocity. Erickson illustrated the dynamic, stating; "Now what can I do and what can you do? First I do this and then you do that" (Erickson, 1966). According to Erickson, "You very seldom give orders because you do not want the other person to be a helpless slave. You get less labor out of slaves than you do out of free workers." Because the relationship is not characterized by control or dominance, there are times when the patient will yield to the therapist and times when the therapist will yield to the patient (Erickson, 1966).

Paradoxically, one of the problems with seeking to control the patient is that this effort ultimately weakens the position of the therapist. Therapeutic efficacy is predicated on a relationship of trust. If patients do not have trust, or they fear sanctions for revealing their true wishes, then there is little to keep them engaged in the therapeutic effort. While the government's judicial control can be imposed on individuals, regardless of their will, therapeutic influence is founded instead on voluntary compliance (Horwitz, 1982, p. 126). Thus "involuntary therapy" is a contradiction in terms. Although coercion can change conduct, it does not initiate a process of inner healing.

For these reasons, the clinician must always be on guard for situations that might create subtle control battles. Whenever the patient does not respond as the practitioner thinks necessary, there is the temptation to try still harder for the desired result. If a battle for control develops, energy is diverted from the healing process and opportunity is lost for the patient's discovery of inner resources and unrecognized capacities. Toward the end of his career, Erickson was asked what experience had taught him about being a better therapist. He responded by saying that he continually strove to be less controlling (Erickson and Rossi, 1981). Similarly, in numerous lectures during the 1950s and 1960's, Erickson would say, "You must remember that it is not you who is the important one [in healing]: it is the patient." Erickson further clarifies the issue while explaining his work in a specific case, "The burden of responsibility was hers, the means was hers" (Erickson, 1964/2001b, p. 26).

While seeking to provide assistance to those who were suffering, Erickson clearly understood that therapeutic progress depended on the will of the patient. He would often admit that, when he offered help, he was not entirely certain what the patient would do with it. His hope was that the collaboration would lead to useful action. Erickson reminds us that the practitioner should, "always let patients follow their own spontaneous way of doing things" (Erickson, 1962b). In this way, discovery of previously unrecognized capacities and inner resources is better facilitated and control battles are avoided.

No matter what the patient does in response to the therapeutic stimulus, another opportunity for engaging the patient is presented. When a change of direction is needed, the practitioner must appeal to preexisting motivational forces within the patient. An analogy can be drawn from tennis. When the racquet receives an incoming ball it has no control over the direction or velocity of the incoming object. However, the racket can be tilted slightly up or slightly down and the ball will react in a very different manner. To direct the ball properly, the focus of control is on the racket's surface and not the properties of the tennis ball. Whenever possible, patients are to be treated within the office as acting appropriately regardless of the behavior they display.

In the case of Johnny's wet bed, Erickson did not attempt to make Johnny stop the behavior. Instead he shifted the focus of attention to Johnny's accomplishments. These were accomplishments that represented the goodness of his body. This tilted the situation in such a way that Johnny's normal and natural development enabled him to grow out of problem. While describing this case, Erickson explained, "I told him *WE* would have to wait and see when he would have his first dry bed" (Erickson, 1964a). This was how Erickson situationally defined everyone's role in the healing process. It was not Erickson's job to tell Johnny what to do. He instead created a general expectation of success, a structure of belief on which Johnny could hang any personal goal. No matter how Johnny responded, Erickson would achieve his goal as long as Johnny achieved some sense of accomplishment.

All of Erickson's problem solving efforts were characterized by a focus on the growth of the individual. As a parent, Erickson showed the same appreciation for personal goals as he showed as a clinician. His style as a father was to offer possibilities and to support individual growth as he encouraged each child to find their own path of success. As a highly revered mentor, he refused to indoctrinate students with his way of doing therapy but instead promoted the same process of continual growth and self-discovery by which his own life was characterized.

Yet, man is not an island unto himself. Erickson taught that each individual is an integral part of society, both contributing to it and receiving from it. Opportunities for change can take place in the psychological, behavioral, biological, or social milieu and these changes impact all other aspects of the individual life experience. It is not important in which arena change is initiated. Erickson's interventions frequently involved activities that made use of or capitalized on connections in some, many, or all arenas. As Erickson demonstrated, when a relationship is perceived as mutually beneficial, then the impetus of cooperation can be capitalized on.

Chapter 5

A Philosophical Framework

This chapter makes use of philosophical terms that did not come from Erickson's writing or lectures, but that provide a philosophical background for understanding his clinical construction of hope. An important question to be answered in this chapter is, "How can patients turn to someone outside of themselves for help and yet retain the integrity of their personal will?" While striving to avoid the use of unnecessary jargon, the terms used in this chapter are meant to act as coordinates to help locate Erickson's position in relation to other celebrated thinkers.

Case report: The woman with Raynaud's disease

A 50-year-old woman diagnosed with Raynaud's disease, came into Erickson's office in a state of extreme pain and sleep deprivation. She showed her hands to Erickson and said, "I have got ulcerated fingers from lack of circulation to my hands. I have already had one finger amputated and now expect to have another amputation." She described her pain as being so intense that she could only sleep for one or two hours at a time.

Erickson responded by saying that he did not know much about treating Raynaud's disease. He told her that if there were anything that could be done about this, her own "body learnings" would take care of the matter. He taught her how to go into a trance, during which he explained she had a tremendous amount of body learning, the visceral abilities that we all accumulate over a lifetime of experience. He suggested that during the day, her unconscious mind be completely absorbed in correlating all of her body learnings to use for her benefit. Before going to bed, she was to sit in a chair and develop a trance state and during that trance she was to put all of her learnings into action. After coming out of that trance, she was to call Erickson.

The woman followed Erickson's prescribed routine. Before bed-time she went into a trance. She called Erickson at 10:30 p.m. and in a trembling voice said, "My husband is holding the phone because I am too weak to hold the receiver. I am scared! I can scarcely sit in the chair. I did exactly what you said. I sat in the chair and went into a trance and then all of a sudden I started to get cold. I got colder and colder, just like when I was a little girl in Minnesota. I shrived all over for about twenty minutes. My teeth even chattered! Then all of a sudden the cold disappeared and I began to get warm. I felt burning hot all over! Now I have devel-oped a profound sense of physical relaxation and fatigue."

Erickson responded by saying, "Congratulations for teaching me how to handle this sort of a problem. Now go to bed and call me when you wake up." Erickson received the next call at 8 a.m. It was her first continuous night's sleep in over ten years.

Erickson explained this success by saying, "I did not do anything other than to tell her to utilize, in her own way, her own special body learnings." Several months later he received a letter telling him that she had remained free of pain by using this method of capillary dilation in her arms, wrists, and hands. Each night, before she went to bed, she would alter the circulation of her blood so that she was able to achieve comfort in her hands and was there-fore able to sleep through the night.

(Erickson, 1960a)

A fundamental characteristic underlying all of Erickson's teaching and therapy is his *deep respect for the individuality of each person.* During his clinical work he was careful to create therapeutic space for patients to accomplish their objectives, *in their own way.* Erickson did not believe patients should be made to conform to other people's theoretical models of change. He believed that *the philosophy of change must come from the patient* and not from the textbook.

Erickson refused to endorse any single goal for therapy and did not believe that any of the existing schools of psychotherapy could properly consider the totality of each individual's uniqueness (Erickson-Elliott, and Erickson-Klein, 1991). His *unique* approach has been described as non-directive; however, this term is deceiving because it implies a passive rather than active role for the therapist. As can be seen in the preceding case report, Erickson was more proactive than passive. He worked in a strategic manner and did not simply wait for problems to resolve themselves (Haley, 1973).

In psychotherapy, a strategic approach typically involves an assessment of the patient's belief about the problem and the creation of a healing ritual that is presented in a manner as consistent as possible with the patient's belief system (Fish, 1973). This practice has been further refined within the context of the client-directed approach, which seeks to continually evaluate and re-align the direction of therapy to match the patient's meanings and preferences (Duncan, Miller and Sparks, 2004, p. 192). A great deal of Erickson's skill was in knowing how to help people recognize and achieve their own personal goals. In fact, that was his primary objective.

Erickson's approach can be described as a meta-teleology. The word "teleology" is a philosophical term used to describe the study of purpose and its byproduct, goal setting. A *teleological* perspective recognizes people's efforts to find direction in life by looking to some end. The term "meta" is a prefix used to describe something that exists outside of a single point of reference. It encompasses every possibility within a given field. Therefore, when a person makes it his purpose to help others establish meaningful goals, of their own design, then a meta-teleological approach exists. This is the philosophical term that comes closest to describing the therapeutic objective described in this text.

Erickson's creative use of hypnosis challenged the traditional notion that the ultimate objective of all hypnotic techniques is suggestion. In the type of hypnosis he pioneered, the utilization of general human tendencies and individual characteristics becomes the primary focus. In Ericksonian therapy, all problem-solving strategies are inextricably linked to recognition and promotion of the patient's will. In this meta-teleology, suggestions, inspiration, and encouragement serve as mechanisms for activating internal resources. *A clinical breakthrough occurs whenever patients gain a new appreciation for what they can do.*

In the case of the woman with Raynaud's disease, the catalyst was encouragement from a medical expert, Erickson. This enabled her to understand that she had an enormous number of previously unrecognized learnings and that these visceral learnings could be used to achieve her objectives.

There is a powerful healing energy, produced by the combination of hope and utility, that results in greater resiliency. In order to maintain health, patients need to recognize that there is some meaningful thing that can be done in relation to their problems. Without a reason to act, there is no initiative. As shown from numerous studies on positive expectancy, hope produces symptom relief and promotes physical healing. Such studies have shown that placebo treatments, which are one means of producing hope, lessen the severity of arthritis, reduce the frequency of asthma attacks, relieve hay fever, suppress coughs, alleviate tension and anxiety, cure headaches, reduce pain, prevent colds, cure ulcers, inhibit symptoms of withdrawal from narcotics, alter gastric functioning, control the blood sugar levels of diabetics, reduce enuresis, reduce the frequency and severity of angina attacks, and reverse the growth of malignant tumors (Beecher, 1961; Honigfeld, 1964; Klopfer, 1957; Volgyesi, 1954). In contrast, negative emotional states increase vulnerability to physical disease, aggravate existing illness, and retard the process of healing (Frank, 1973). Thus, hopefulness not only encourages symptomatic relief but also appears to promote physical healing.

A resilient response to problem situations emanates from a belief in the innate goodness of self. Without a healthy self-appreciation, people either position their energy against the self (e.g. someone who starves the body because of anorexia) or, at the very least, are unable to summon their resources. Erickson made it clear that his objective was to communicate the goodness and soundness of the patient's body. According to Erickson, patients need a feeling of security in their own body (Erickson, 1962c). When convinced of the goodness of the mind, heart, digestive system, or any other part of the body that has been psychologically disenfranchised, a new sense of self-efficacy is created.

A similar point has been made by Jefferson Fish (1973) who argued (p. 17):

The important point is that the patient must be persuaded that it is what *he* does, not what the therapist does, which results in his being cured. This belief is crucial because it implies that the patient is the master of his behavior rather than its servant.

As suggested by contemporary research, the secret to resiliency is a sense of control over what has been happening during a moment of trial (Bandura, 2003). This sense of personal ability enables patients to employ inner capacities and experiential learnings to achieve their objectives.

Another important element highlighted by the case of the woman with Raynaud's disease, was Erickson's instruction for her to trust her unconscious mind. This gave her a sense of utility and gave her hope. She was directed toward the goodness of her own mental resources. In contrast to Freud's ideas about the unconscious mind, Erickson always emphasized the goodness of the patient's unconscious mind. He often used this construct to communicate the idea that patients have within themselves a yet unrecognized force that can be trusted and relied upon, something that holds much more potential than can ever be fully known. This was the type of encouragement that characterized his approach.

Although there may be numerous objectives that are pursued during the course of psychotherapy, there should always be a single clinical objective that provides a navigational point. Similar to a beacon on a high mountain, this overarching objective allows the practitioner to navigate around various obstacles while maintaining a sense of direction. The objective is the pinnacle point that justifies all other subordinate goals. Within the context of Ericksonian therapy, *the primary objective behind all psychotherapeutic endeavors is to stimulate the activation of unrecognized abilities for purposes determined by the will of the patient.* This is the meta-teleology of change.

"All that we do is done with an eye to something else."
– Aristotle, 384–322 BCE

Summary

As we study the philosophy behind Erickson's approach to healing, it should be apparent that therapy is an opportunity for the patient and therapist to do something meaningful in relation to the patient's needs. The direction in which these energies will be employed is determined by the will of the patient rather than some external doctrine of change. The goal of the therapist is to strategically promote the health-oriented goals of the patient.[1] In this way, therapy *does not* take on a spirit of coercion, superiority, or indoctrination, but instead is characterized by a process of mutual learning and discovery.

In the way that a physician can choose from many types of medication, therapy can be achieved using an endless variety of psychological processes, activated by an equally wide variety of techniques. The clinical strategies from which these techniques are derived should not be viewed as a curative agent but instead as a means of boosting the psychological immune system and stimulating an internal healing process. Thus, emphasis is placed on the inner capacities of the patient rather than the actions of the therapist. Lastly, perfectionistic goals and egotistical ideas are to be avoided. Rather than think, "I must find a solution to this problem," it was Erickson's approach to think in terms of the patient's resiliency and hope for the future.

---

[1] For every rule there is an expectation. Some patients have goals that are unrealistic or self-destructive, so this is not a point of therapeutic engagement. But almost all human beings have at least one goal that is health-oriented and worthy of support.

Part II

Clinical Strategies

Chapter 6

Introduction to the Six Core Strategies

Distraction: Unintentional progress impedes self-sabotage.

Partitioning: When everything cannot be made right, it is good to have something that is rectified.

Progression: It is not possible to cure every sickness but there is always some good that can be done for those who suffer.

Suggestion: All problem solving begins with the idea that change is possible.

Reorientation: The greater the complexity of a person's psychological problem, the greater opportunity to discover a simple solution.

Utilization: Whenever you try to *make* a person change, you encourage animosity, but, if you offer an opportunity, your energy is not wasted.

These six statements reflect some of the most important lessons taught by Milton Erickson. These axioms briefly illustrate the functional definition of everything that is to follow in the coming text. Although the wording is from Dan Short, the ideas are drawn from one of the most legendary figures in the field of psychiatry and psychology.

The master of a craft, one who is exceedingly accomplished at complex tasks, has the ability to apply robust strategies in order to quickly solve problems. Once a skill has become practiced to the point of automaticity, it requires less and less conscious deliberation and is more likely to occur as a spontaneous response. So, efficiency is greatly increased, as each conscious decision represents numerous chains of implicit reasoning. This is one reason veteran clinicians often have difficulty articulating the clinical strategies they employ. Their responses have become so practiced that to deliberate consciously on each step would only cause them to falter.

Within the context of psychotherapeutics, what has commonly been referred to as "clinical intuition" is more accurately understood as implicit reason. This distinguishes it as a logical process that is distinctly different from creative guessing or "luck." Individuals seeking to acquire problem solving skills, such as Erickson had, benefit from having the enigmatic strategies of a genius made clear.

Part II of this book has been designed to elaborate on several of Erickson's strategies for clinical problem solving. As with a skeleton key, each strategy can be applied to a variety of problem situations in order to arrive at new and unique solutions. What will become apparent is that the broader the application of a particular strategy, the more uses that can be made of it.

A clinical strategy is simply defined as a fundamental principle of human problem solving. Clinical strategies allow expert clinicians to design specialized techniques to address a wide variety of emotional and psychological challenges. In order to know the difference between a technique and a strategy, it should be recognized that distinct psychotherapeutic techniques, such as double bind, symptom prescription, and paradoxical directive, can be grouped into categories that illustrate some common function. It is this functional understanding of technique that allows the practitioner to operate in a strategic fashion. This is one reason why it is so important to develop an understanding of the strategies that govern a class of techniques. When a practitioner blindly applies a therapeutic technique, without fully understanding the clinical function, resourcefulness is impeded and success becomes random.

An understanding of clinical strategies fosters less dependency on predetermined procedures and greater use of clinical judgment. Although clinical judgment has been almost universally accepted as an essential factor in psychotherapeutics, very few therapies provide a means of teaching it. While describing the problem of automated responses in therapy, Erickson (1977/2001, p. 3) explained,

> In therapeutic approaches, one must always take into considera-
> tion the actual personality of the individual ... Are they over-
> friendly? hostile? defiant? extroverted? introverted? ... the
> therapist must be fairly fluid in his behavior, because if he is rigid
> he is going to elicit certain types of rigid behavior in the patient.

This is not a text about therapeutic techniques. There are no rigid step-by-step formulae to be memorized and applied in each therapy session. The goal of this book is much more ambitious. In the way that Erickson was able to design a new technique for almost every new case, the following clinical strategies provide a basis for fluid clinical judgment. Although each chapter contains a series of techniques used by Erickson and others, these behavioral proto-cols are not to be blindly mimicked. Each therapy situation requires sufficient clinical judgment to design or modify tech-niques in order to meet a multitude of unique clinical variables.

Within the context of healing, powerful and sophisticated psy-chotherapeutics rarely involve a single clinical strategy. It is instead a skillful combination of procedures that together promote the idea that change is possible. While it seems obvious that effec-tive therapies must offer more than one technique, not much con-sideration has been given to the number of strategies afforded by each school of therapy. It is difficult to find another single approach to psychotherapy that incorporates as many strategies for healing as the Ericksonian approach. There are at least six strategic positions that emerge from Erickson's work. These are *distraction, partitioning, progression, suggestion, reorientation,* and *utilization.*

These strategies are by no means mutually exclusive. They can be thought of as primary colors. Each can be arranged and mixed with others in order to create wide-ranging yet highly precise responses to a given problem. A very nice example of this can be seen in some creative problem solving by Erickson for two of his children. At the time, Roxanna Erickson-Klein was only five and she had been injured by her big brother, Lance. He accidentally caught her foot in the bottom of a door tearing the nail from her big toe. Roxanna was hurt not only by the physical injury but also by the fact that her brother did not seem sufficiently remorseful for what he had done.

After the physical wound was cared for, Erickson brought Roxanna into his office and carefully explained to her that if Lance would lift her up onto his shoulders, she would find a secret "off/on switch" on the ceiling. Roxanna was instructed not to tell Lance what she was looking for but that, once she had it, she was free to install and operate it in whatever manner she chose. Roxanna went to her brother and he cheerfully complied with her request to be on his shoulders. Roxanna found the imaginary switch without difficulty, but then could not decide whether it should be installed inside or outside her clothing. Not only did Roxanna's toe stop bothering her, she also felt uplifted by her brother and was no longer as sore over the incident (Erickson-Klein, 1990, p. 284). This illustrates the way in which highly individualized procedures defy replication in the form of a general technique. It is absolutely absurd to imagine using the "piggy-back" technique with every patient who presents with an injured toe.

However, when this case is viewed as a combination of two strategies, distraction and reorientation, it begins to make more sense. While looking for the imaginary switch, Roxanna was distracted from her pain. Once she found this prized object, she was further distracted by the task of having to decide where to install it and how it should be operated. The fundamental reorientation was that she discovered new possibilities for gaining control over her pain and over her brother. She was no longer in a "one-down" position in relation to her brother. Furthermore, Lance was able to resolve his own feelings of guilt by doing his sister a favor and being a part of an intervention that was intended to help her feel better. When this series of events is understood at this level, then the functional elements can be strategically replicated using an unlimited number of variations.

As with the first part of the book, each strategy will be introduced with a case report. Rather than have the case explained immediately afterward, the reader is encouraged to ponder the clinical narrative while reading the description of the fundamental principle and its general applications. The question to ask is, "Why did Erickson do it that way?" Each overview is filled with detailed elaborations and additional case examples illustrating numerous techniques that serve a common function. Toward the end of each section, attention is turned back toward the introductory case example and analysis is provided. The last section in each chapter contains general principles that serve as guidelines for a variety of clinical situations. The content in these chapters is not meant to be memorized as a sort of stale doctrine but rather to serve as a spark for imagination and continued discovery.

Chapter 7

Distraction

This chapter describes a strategy most often used for coping with pain. However, any health-related endeavor that causes intense fear, such as an impending surgery, requires some strategy for gaining the cooperation of the patient. This is especially true for psychotherapy. As stated by Erickson (1977a), "The secret of psychotherapy lies in getting the patient to do something they want to do but ordinarily would not." Essentially, this is what the chapter is about.

Case report: The old gentleman who was scared of elevators

An elderly gentleman came to Erickson for help with a longstanding fear of elevators. He had worked at the top of a tall building for many years and had always had to walk up using the stairs. However, this solution became less feasible as he became older. Erickson knew this was a prudish man who was married to a prudish wife. After listening to him ask if he could be helped with his fear of elevators, Erickson confidently responded, "I will probably scare the pants off you, in another direction." The man responded that nothing could be worse than his fear of an elevator.

This was during the 1940s, when elevators had operators. In this man's building, the operators were young females. Erickson met in advance with one of the attendants in order to make special arrangements. She agreed to cooperate and thought Erickson's idea sounded as though it would be fun. The following day, Erickson escorted the gentleman to the office building. As the man had explained earlier, he was not afraid of walking into the elevator but when it began to move the experience became unbearable. So Erickson had him practice going in and out of an elevator. Then at a moment when both Erickson and the man were fully inside, Erickson told the girl to close the door and said, "Let's go up." She took the elevator up one story and stopped it between two floors.

The man began to yell, "What's wrong?" Erickson said, "The elevator girl wants to kiss you." Shocked, the gentleman said, "But I
am a married man!" The girl said, "I don't mind that." She walked
toward him. He stepped back and said, "You start the elevator!" So
she started it. She went up to the fourth floor and stopped again
between floors. She said, "I just have a craving for a kiss." He said,
"You go on about your business." He wanted the elevator moving,
not standing still. She replied, "Well, let's go down and start all
over again." And she began to take the elevator down. He said,
"Not down, up!" as he did not want to go through that all over
again. She started the elevator and then stopped between floors
again and said, "Do you promise that you will ride down in my
elevator with me when you are through with work?" He said, "I'll
promise anything if you will promise not to kiss me." From then
on he was able to ride without fear, of the elevator.

(Haley, 1973, pp. 297–9)

Perhaps one of the most successful messages in recent times is the
Nike advertising slogan, "Just do it." This brief imperative provides an answer for difficult moments when one is faced with
extraordinary demands. Although we typically prefer to know in
advance *how to do* what must be done, novel accomplishments
require learning that comes primarily from doing. How else could
the explorers Lewis and Clark know how to cross from end to end
of an uncharted continent? The first step was to do it. Similarly,
how is the therapy patient going to know how to live his or her life
in an entirely different manner without first doing it? Yet in clinical practice it is not uncommon to encounter individuals who have
become paralyzed by fear and are unwilling to risk unfamiliar
behavior. So how do you help a person who will not *just do it*? The
answer is to keep their eyes and mind set on something else. The
basic premise is similar to having a person, who fears heights but
must cross a high bridge, look somewhere else other than down. It
should be recognized that it is not the distraction of vision that is
most essential: it is instead the distraction of the mind from overwhelming thoughts.

The clinical strategy of distraction can be defined as a temporary
separation of thought and action resulting in a greater dependency
on highly automated behavioral patterns. While the body is

engaged in one important task, the mind is focused on another. Perhaps the most common example of this natural behavior is the automobile driver who travels from his home to the office without any conscious recollection of how he got there. His mind was distracted by other pressing issues while his body responded automatically to cues and navigated the car safely through traffic.

Distraction is a strategy that is particularly useful for counteracting the effects of self-fulfilling prophecies or highly conditioned responses to feared stimuli. Perhaps the most classic example is the frightened child (or adult) who must receive medicine by injection. Just the sight of the needle is enough to produce hypersensitivity in the nerves and hypertension in the muscles. A child might even attempt to escape, thereby resulting in restraint, which increases the fear of the situation as it turns into a vicious cycle. The end result is a dramatic increase in the amount of pain experienced by the child and subsequent trauma. However when the child is told to look at a bowl of candy and decide which color he wants, and the needle is kept out of sight, it is possible the small prick might go undetected. During his residency, Erickson developed a clever method of distraction for similar situations. As the patient sat waiting for the painful medical procedure Erickson would comment, "I just hope you don't get that slow-poke nurse. It will be so much less painful if you get the nurse with the quick hands." In this way the patient's attention was entirely distracted by who the nurse was and how Erickson responded to her arrival. Did he seem relieved? If so, the patient could relax and just wonder how painful it would have been if he would have gotten the wrong nurse (Erickson, 1966).

In regard to psychological distress, there are many conditions that become chronic or worsen over time due to the effects of self-fulfilling prophecy. Any time the patient strongly anticipates a negative outcome, this expectation alone may sustain symptomatic behaviors that would have otherwise diminished. An example is the spiraling effect created by the person who is so nervous that he will stutter during conversation that he can hardly speak. Another example is the young child with asthma who becomes so fearful of having another attack that he tenses all the muscles in his chest, leaving hardly any room for the inflation of the lungs. A common scenario with depression is that patients begin to experience feelings of hopelessness or worthlessness and respond by staying in bed all day, or watching TV for twelve straight hours, or finishing off a bottle of vodka. These behaviors make them feel even worse about themselves, thus feeding the cycle of depression: "What a wretched person I am!" In each of these cases, the self-perpetuating cycle can be interrupted when the person is distracted by an activity that is somehow incompatible with the negative expectancy. Whenever a negative expectancy is left unfulfilled, more energy is available for new learning.[1]

In the case mentioned above, the man's fear of elevators was most likely based on the discomfort generated by the total situation. He had always avoided elevators, and was probably not accustomed to the internal sensations created by the sudden upward movement. He was also a "proper" gentleman and probably not accustomed to being a passenger in a vehicle driven by a young female. Being alone in a small space with a young woman might have also been very uncomfortable for him. As emphasized by Erickson, he was not afraid to walk in and out of the elevator, nor was he afraid of having his office on a top floor. This is why upward movement was the subject of treatment rather than the problem of claustrophobia or fear of heights. Considering that every one of the elevator attendants was a young female, it is interesting that Erickson initially said, "I will probably scare the pants off you, in another direction." If the elevator is going up, and that is what he is currently afraid of, the only other direction would be down. In this way Erickson foreshadowed the use of an intervention that in some way would involve sexual innuendo. By having the elevator operator threaten to kiss the fearful man, his attention was suddenly drawn to her lips and away from any sensations in his own body. Furthermore, he was no longer as concerned with the space between his feet and the ground floor as he was with the space between him and the young woman. The distraction was practically irresistible and, as a result, new meaning was given to the *rise* in that *old elevator*.

---

[1] This idea is explained in greater detail in Chapter 10, in the section on Confusion.

Red herring

Case report: The girl who could not bear to be watched

A girl with tremendous anxiety came to Phoenix to receive therapy from Erickson. Her behavior was extremely rigid and limiting. She had rituals around dressing. It had to be done in a certain way. She had a rigid ritual for reading her mail. She would sit only on certain objects. She would live only in a certain apartment. And she had a constant compulsion to clean herself. On some days she would spend as long as 19 hours bathing.

According to Erickson, "One of the first things I did to her was to let her tell me what utterly, utterly intense anxiety she had while trying to get herself clean." During this conversation the girl tried to convince Erickson that she was completely absorbed in this tremendous anxiety. He had her tell her story at length and, as soon as she had convinced herself that the anxiety was so awful that she could be aware of nothing else, he agreed with her. With great curiosity he then asked, "As absorbed as you will be in this awful, awful, anxiety, while showering, you will not mind if I watch you." He described her reaction to the statement has being greatly jarred, "… practically loose from her teeth!"

It should be clear that Erickson had not said that he would do such a thing. He merely asked a curious question to expand her rigid perspective. But she did not want to even speculate on the possibility. She was forced to admit that she just could not tolerate such a thing. Erickson argued her previous position: "Surely you will be so absorbed in your anxiety that you will not know anyone is there." At this point her anxiety over showering no longer seemed so absorbing.

Next, Erickson pointed out, "Really, it is not so bad that you would be so absorbed in your anxiety that you would be unaware of someone watching you. In fact, I would be willing to bet that I could just rattle the door to the bathroom and you would notice it." Then Erickson pointed out that just wondering if he would come over and rattle it would be enough to keep her distracted from what she had previously perceived as inescapable anxiety.

(Erickson, 1958e)

The expression "red herring" comes from the practice of a hunted man drawing this type of fish across his trail in order to distract hounds. In therapy, emotionally charged decoys can be used to distract the patient so that the focus of attention is narrowed and kept from otherwise overwhelming aspects of the situation.

Erickson often explained this technique using examples from dentistry. Many of his patients were terrified of a trip to the dentist, especially if a syringe was going to be used. So Erickson would advise the dentist to have the patient sitting in such a position that he could see the tray holding a big, long needle. When the dentist entered the room his statement was, "I will use hypnosis first and that should block the pain. But if you start to become uncomfortable, then we can use that shot over there." The needle is the red herring that distracts the patient from what the dentist is doing to the teeth (Erickson, 1962c).

The case at the beginning of this section provides a beautiful example of how distraction can be carried out on multiple levels. In having the girl describe her bathing habits, Erickson was initiating a process of systematic desensitization. The girl did not resist the procedure because she did not recognize it. She forgot to become self-conscious while talking about herself being in the nude because she was so distracted by her need to convince Erickson of how much anxiety she experienced *while bathing*. By the time she realized that she was causing a man to speculate on her bathing behavior, something associated with nakedness, it was too late. The only way out of the situation was to convince him that her anxiety was not so tremendous and that she would certainly notice anyone watching her.

As she shifted gears and began to argue Erickson's therapeutic message, he was able to further weaken the strength of the anxiety by reinforcing and expanding her new line of debate (i.e. "I am not *that* anxious"). It should be noted that it was Erickson's integrity and respect for the patient that made this intervention successful. If the patient had suspected she was being propositioned sexually, the results would have been disastrous. What is missing from this brief account is a detailed account of Erickson's rapport building and creation of a safe environment for therapy.

Questioning and presupposition

Case report: The homicidal patient in the elevator

While working at a psychiatric hospital late in the night, Erickson found himself suddenly trapped in a dangerous situation. A homicidal patient had hidden himself in an elevator and Erickson did not see him until after he had stepped in and slammed the door shut. It locked automatically and, although Erickson had a key to unlock it, he did not have the time needed to escape. The homicidal patient serenely stated, "I've been waiting for you to make the evening rounds. Every one is down at the other end of the ward and I am going to kill you." Erickson's statement was just as simple, "Well, are you going to do the slaughter right there … or over there?" The patient looked at the first spot Erickson had chosen and then at the second. As he did this, Erickson opened the door and said, "Of course, there is a chair over there that you could sit in afterwards … that is true you know. And at the same time there is a chair down there." And as he spoke, Erickson began walking. "And there is another chair over there and another spot at the other end of the corridor." The patient walked along with Erickson looking at each spot that he could pick for Erickson's demise. Eventually they arrived at the station where the attendants were gathered.

(Erickson, 1959c)

One of the most effective means of creating an immediate distraction is to ask a question. Questions are highly distracting and usually compel the person to think about what has been asked. In fact, most people have become conditioned to the idea that they must think about and answer questions once they are asked. This is why sales people are trained to respond to resistance with a complex series of questions. The mantra taught to sales trainees is, "The person asking the questions is the person who is in control of the conversation."

The term *presupposition* is used to describe a linguistic maneuver in which one statement presupposes the validity of another. Although presupposition can occur without the use of questions, it works especially well with implied meanings hidden beneath the surface of the question. For instance the question, "Are you aware of the progress you have made during this first visit?" obviously implies that progress has been made, yet the patient's attention is distracted by the question of awareness. The question, "Will you be ready to get over that habit this week or the next?" can also be viewed as a double bind (Erickson, Rossi, and Rossi, 1976, p. 65). However, essentially the question acts as distraction from the other less desirable thought, "I might never recover." When faced with an interesting question, one that seems meaningful or important, patients are likely to focus on their answer rather than on the underlying implications. Questions that focus the attention on the issue of time contain a strong psychological implication that the desired outcome will be achieved (Erickson, Rossi, and Rossi, 1976).

As a rule, more power is added to the method of distraction when emotions are involved. When necessary, Erickson would ask a seemingly rude or embarrassing question to further distract from the statement's implied meaning. As Erickson would explain, "Before the patient goes in for that dangerous medical procedure you ask her if she would be willing to send you the recipe for son-of-a-gun stew once she gets home. And you can explain how much you love son-of-a-gun stew." While the patient may be a little put off by the doctor's self-centeredness at this moment of crisis in her life, she does not consciously recognize the implication that there is absolute certainty that she will recover and go home from the hospital (Erickson, 1966). It is difficult to reject a statement that you do not know you have accepted. Using the same technique Erickson would speculate out loud with a patient about recovery from enuresis, "Will you have your first dry bed on Monday, Tuesday, or Friday? Surely, Sunday of this week is too soon." The distraction of naming the day leads the patient away from the unhappy thought of never having a dry bed. In other instances of implying the inevitable success of therapy, Erickson would state, "I do not know if our last visit will be before or after the spring." In this way the patient is distracted by the suspense of unanswered questions and yet retains the freedom to choose the outcome.

When done in the proper manner, distraction is not used as a trick but instead as an avenue to a legitimate therapeutic objective.

When the homicidal patient made his statement to Erickson, he undoubtedly wanted to be taken seriously. As Erickson explains, "I accepted the idea that the patient was going to kill me." Then, with his statement accepted, the patient was free to search for an answer to Erickson's questions. And what else did the questioning allow the patient to do? He was now in a position to tell the psychiatrist *where to go*. If we assume that his basic agenda was to be taken seriously by a significant authority figure, then his mission was accomplished. As Erickson might ask us, "Why not use the patient's attitude?" Explaining his work with this patient Erickson states, "You accept their thinking. You never try to fight it. You never tangle with it. You simply utilize it for elaborating and extending the patient's thinking in every helpful way" (Erickson, 1959c).

Emphasis on detail

Case report: Allan's bleeding leg

While playing outside, Erickson's seven-year-old son, Allan, fell on a broken bottle and slashed his leg open. Allan came into the house screaming. His leg was bleeding profusely. When Allan paused to get a breath for the next scream, Erickson gave a very urgent instruction, "Get a *big* towel, Allan. Not the small one. Get a *big* towel … a *big* towel!" After Allan accomplished that, Erickson instructed him, "For heaven's sakes, wrap it tightly. Not loosely. Wrap it tightly! Wrap it tightly!" After Allan finished wrapping his leg Erickson was able to approve of the good job he had done. The towel was nice and tight and Allan was no longer crying.

Before taking him to the surgeon, Erickson prepared Allan by telling him what he should do. When Allan walked into the surgeon's office he boldly stated, "I want 100 stitches! My sister is always bragging about the stitches that she has got and I want more than she has!" The surgeon got him on the examining table, looked over the leg and asked Erickson, "General anesthetic?" Erickson casually commented, "Listen to Allan. He will tell you what he wants." So Allan patiently explained again to the surgeon that he wanted 100 stitches. The surgeon washed his leg and started suturing, without any anesthesia. Allan was not complaining about pain. Instead he admonished the surgeon, "Wait a minute. Not so far apart. Put them closer together." The surgeon looked at Allan in disbelief as he held his leg up and insisted that he get more stitches. Throughout the rest of the procedure Allan looked at what was being done, and he supervised, and he criticized.

(Erickson, 1955b)

Most people have had the experience of being so completely absorbed in a complex task that there was no attention left to consider other immediate circumstances. If a task is important enough and it requires close attention to detail, other competing stimuli are ignored. In the case of Erickson's son, Allan, it was the pain and fear of injury that was shut out as Allan listened carefully to the detailed instructions coming from his father. Erickson did not want Allan to think about his hurting, or be worried about the bleeding. But he did want him involved in doing something about the problem. Allan became focused on getting exactly the right size of towel and on wrapping it correctly. Thus the technique of distraction simultaneously created an opportunity for competency building. While at the surgeon's office, Allan's primary concern was getting as many stitches as possible. Erickson had initiated this thinking by telling him that he should, "Put an end to Betty Alice's bragging about how many stitches she had." As Erickson explains, "All I did was redirect Allan's attention to one small aspect of his experience." Erickson had also encouraged Allan to pay attention to the details of the surgeon's work to meet his goal of outdoing his sister.

When a person is given very precise and detailed instructions with a strong emotional emphasis on detail, there is a tendency to focus on how to respond. Less attention is given to the possibility of not responding at all. When used correctly, this type of distraction enables the patient to approach a difficult therapeutic task with greater determination. For this reason distraction is typically used to counterbalance strong stimuli that would otherwise distract from therapy, such as physical pain, fear, and anxiety.

When considering the broad application of this strategy it is important to recognize what portion of reality should be given more attention as well as what portion should be distracted from.

Therapy can be dichotomized as having one of two possible out-comes—either success or failure. Common sense and everyday experience tell us that success is more likely when it is the focus of attention. People who start to give too much attention to their own shortcomings tend to perform less well. In sports, this is com-monly called "choking." In therapy it is referred to as "self-fulfill-ing prophecy." Therapists should create a positive self-fulfilling prophecy by elaborating on desired or productive therapeutic pos-sibilities rather than on the hazards of failing to change. This does not mean that the therapist has to avoid discussion of possible negative consequences: rather the opposite is true. The complete avoidance of a topic forces the patient to do his own speculation without the help of informed guidance. However, while address-ing both sides of an issue, it makes sense to elaborate more fully on the side that will be the more beneficial once it is recognized as a new possibility for the patient.

Therapeutic amnesia

Case report: The woman who watched where she sat

A woman entered Erickson's office and hesitated before sitting down. She studied each chair in the room to make certain that she did not sit in the wrong chair. This was her presenting problem. She had to avoid sitting in certain types of chairs. She was exceed-ingly compulsive about this issue. Wherever she went she had to examine chairs carefully. Not only did she feel overly self-con-scious, but she was also prevented from enjoying the freedom that comes from carefree lounging.

Erickson used hypnosis to communicate the idea of gradually working up to a state of greater and greater freedom from concern. Progression was central to this therapy (the strategy of progression is explained in Chapter 9). However, he was careful to emphasize the importance of hypnotic amnesia—he did not want her to remember his suggestions. She needed to be distracted from the task of becoming more spontaneous, otherwise the progress would be blocked by self-consciousness about spontaneity. She left his office not knowing for certain if any therapy had been accomplished.

One day she happened to notice that she sat down without examining the chair. Then she realized she had been doing this for some time. This caused her to do some thinking and she recognized that she had been going regularly to the movies with a friend, something she had not been able to do for several years. She had also gone to the symphony for the first time in several years. Sometime later, while describing her success to Erickson, she indicated that she never did recognize when she lost the need to examine chairs. According to her understanding, she just automatically began sitting in chairs freely and comfortably.

(Erickson, 1962c)

There are many case examples of Erickson's offering the patient permission to forget things that might detract from therapy. It seems that Erickson used amnesia as a method of distraction when the distraction was needed for several days or weeks. Premature conscious awareness is particularly difficult for patients who suffer from overwhelming childhood trauma or those who have strong competing beliefs that result in acts of self-sabotage. When seen as a strategy of distraction, amnesia becomes a means to *permit the uninhibited development of new learnings* rather than an attempt to permanently erase memories (Gilligan, 1987). Because the strategy of progression requires the passage of time, amnesia is often helpful in this regard as well. Without this complementary intervention the patient might start to lose confidence in therapy. As the saying goes, "A watched pot never boils."

Another common piece of advice is, "Don't think about it so much and the problem will eventually take care of itself." And this is often true. Many problems exist primarily as a byproduct of misguided prevention strategies. This is especially true for those individuals who have developed a neurotic preoccupation that, as a consequence, reinforces the problem behavior. This phenomenon can be understood using the concept of cognitive dissonance. Whenever a great deal of time, energy, or effort is put into something, then that thing has an increase in significance. If you spend several hours a day checking chairs, and do this for many years of your life, then where you sit becomes extremely important, far too important to do in a haphazard way. Then the act of completing the behavior (i.e. sitting safely in a chair) becomes an irresistible reward, thereby causing the cycle to repeat. Conversely, when a person does not invest energy in deciding where to sit, then the choice of chairs is too trivial to deserve attention. Although the solution seems simple, the circular dynamic behind neurotic preoccupations can be difficult to break.

When patients are distracted from nonproductive concerns, there is an increased energy available for other activities. When they pursue rewarding endeavors, not related to problem prevention, a new sense of satisfaction develops. When life feels more rewarding, there is not as much need to seek defense from imagined threats. Rather than live in a world of danger, an individual can experience a world of opportunity.

Hypnotic amnesia is a seemingly complex technique that is sometimes avoided by clinicians out of fear of failure. There is the concern that the suggestion for amnesia will result in the patient's stating, "I remember everything you said"—and it often does. But this response offers yet another opportunity for distraction. Rather than focus on the topic of concern, the clinician can "quiz" the patient in great detail about other benign details of the trance experience. This challenge allows patients to prove their point and thereby maintain a sense of control. If after the second attempt the patient still wants to discuss the ideas that were initially targeted for the amnesia, then the therapist should reconsider the need for distraction. Amnesia is not something to force on another person but is instead an opportunity for the patient to put aside thoughts that are not needed for the task at hand.

Perhaps the most benevolent use of amnesia is in cases of overwhelming distress caused by traumatizing thoughts or memories. By simply being offered permission to forget, the patient is provided with a mechanism by which he or she can temporarily set aside unnerving stimuli. This is a natural behavior which does not require hypnosis. People often act on good opportunities, even without a trance induction. If the person does not like the idea of forgetting about something that has been discussed in therapy, then he or she can simply forget to forget. After all, it is too complicated to remember to forget. And so what is accomplished? Freedom. There is increased freedom whichever way the patient responds.

The general application of distraction

Case report: The boy with severe acne

> A doctor who lived in Massachusetts contacted Erickson and said, "My son's a student at Harvard and he has an extremely bad case of acne. Can you treat that with hypnosis?" Erickson said, "Yes. But why bother bringing him to me? How are you going to spend Christmas vacation?" Her reply was, "I usually take a vacation from medical practice and go to Sun Valley and ski." Erickson said, "Well, this Christmas vacation, why don't you take your son with you? Find a cabin and remove all of the mirrors in it. Eat your meals in the cabin, and be sure that you keep your hand mirror in the safety pocket of your purse." The mother and son spent the vacation time skiing. The young man did not have time to stop and check a mirror. Two weeks later his skin returned to a normal condition.
>
> (Rosen, 1982, p. 87)

Not much needs to be said about the general application of distraction. It is a strategy that is most helpful in cases where the problem is a byproduct of too much attention to temporary life conditions. When there is a frantic attempt to avoid the experience of pain, or intense efforts to avoid having any imperfection in one's beauty, and so on, there is a binding up of one's energy and increased rigidity. When a person becomes entirely oriented toward achieving something that is essentially impossible, the result is a significant decrease in adaptive functioning. This is not true for all psychological issues, however: in some cases the most healing thing the patient can do is to go out and get busy with the business of living and enjoying life. If the person can be distracted long enough, the natural process of change and adaptation can take place.

One note of caution that must be added is that not all forms of distraction are helpful. It is not appropriate to use shocking language or sexual overtures with a patient who feels frightened and vulnerable. The personality of the patient must be carefully studied before one decides on a method of distraction. For example, when Erickson asked his patient if she would notice if he watched her shower, he had carefully considered her needs and tested her response to statements with which she did not agree. With every form of distraction *there must be a degree of safety and trust that is equal to the magnitude of the shock.* As a frail old man confined to a wheelchair, in an office attached to his family home, Erickson was fundamentally safe and could therefore say things that could not be said under different circumstances.

The clinician must not engage in any behavior that is unethical and should also avoid any statement or action that might be mis-interpreted as harassment. The most helpful distractions are those that the patient will eventually look back on with approval and amusement. It is also important to remember that a distraction can be very subtle and still have a profound effect.

In the case example of the boy with acne, it may appear that there is no evidence of treatment. However, this provides an excellent example of recognizing and then facilitating use of the patient's own resources. Erickson's response implied to both the mother and son that the boy already had within him, and within the con-text of his mother's care, all that he needed to heal. Attitude affects virtually every physical condition. Whenever a neurotic complex manifests itself as a dermatological condition, the last thing the patient needs is to feel more self-conscious. So the boy was not given a medical treatment, which would require him to stare into the mirror daily as he applied the medicine. Nor was he told to think positive thoughts, which would require him to reject his nat-ural and spontaneous thoughts. The boy was not told to act in any particular way but instead was met with faith in the goodness of his ability to heal while pleasantly distracted by vacationing with his mother.

Although the outcome in this case may sound somewhat unbe-lievable, the mechanism for recovery is rather simple. Those who have experience with acne know that constant picking or agitation with soaps and astringents causes the skin to produce more oil in an attempt to protect itself from the irritation. When the skin becomes oilier and has more eruptions, the person tends to wash more, thus a vicious cycle is created. Once the skin is left alone, for a period of one to two weeks, it will often heal itself. The only dif-ficulty is in finding a way to distract the person long enough for evidence of improvement to appear. If this distraction technique had not worked for this boy, Erickson would most likely have devised a way to build on the experience and move on to the next type of intervention that common sense would dictate. However, he usually tried the least invasive interventions first, which allowed each person to heal in his or her own way.

Chapter 8

Partitioning

This chapter describes a strategy that helps reduce the emotional impact of an overwhelming life situation. In his lectures, Erickson often used the following case example to illustrate the concept of partitioning. Although it was not his casework, this example nicely illustrates this fundamental strategy. As will be seen in this chapter, there are numerous ways of taking an intolerable situation and breaking it down into smaller, more easily digested parts.

Case report: The hysterical farmer

> A general practitioner in Minnesota had a farmer come running into his office with a broken arm. The arm was bent and the farmer was frightened and hysterical. Rushing around the office he yelled, "You've got to do something for me! You've got to do something for me! You've got to do something for me!" The doctor stepped up to him right away and said, "It hurts pretty bad right there, doesn't it?" The farmer agreed. Next the practitioner said in a soothing voice, "But fortunately it does not hurt down there in your fingers and your shoulder feels all right. It just hurts right there. But not here and not here. Just right there. That's all." Again the farmer had to agree. After a few seconds of having his pain and suffering narrowed down, the farmer became quiet and sat in a chair. His fright and terror was diminished. Next the doctor took care of his arm.

> (Erickson, 1960a; Erickson, 1962c)

For many of those seeking psychotherapeutic care, the duration or complexity of the issues may make the clinical problem seem insurmountable. Healing has not occurred because the available problem-solving resources are overwhelmed and do not seem large enough for the magnitude of the problem. Simply put, there is no feeling of hope. But, like a bundle of sticks, problematic realities can be taken apart so that the full energy of the individual can be brought to bear on a single twig rather than the full bundle. By partitioning the problem, and working on one small fragment at a time, the obstacle is eventually overcome. The same concept is reflected in the well-known military strategy, "divide and conquer." Within the context of psychotherapeutics, it is the clinical problem that is divided, thereby providing the patient with a sense of hope, a feeling that the problem may eventually be conquered.

Partitioning is a broad strategy with almost unlimited applications. It allows the breaking down of negative associations by dividing a boundless problematic reality into smaller, more easily assimilated parts. The strategy was described by Erickson using a variety of terms and has been referenced by some as the fractional approach (Wilson, 2001).

It is also a natural coping strategy that can occur spontaneously for individuals who are overwhelmed, as in the case of severe trauma. Symptomatologies such as depersonalization, amnesia, and dissociation are examples of spontaneous partitions. This is how people protect themselves from stimulus overload. The natural ability to block out some aspects of the total experience becomes a therapeutic strategy when it comes under volitional control. This way it can be used as a tool rather than an involuntary response that intrudes on the tasks of daily living.

An everyday example of healthy and controlled partitioning is reflected in the saying, "I have learned to leave my work at the office." Stressful events that occurred during the work day are partitioned off from events at home with the family. When the person returns to work the next day, the mind recalls all the necessary information associated with this piece of reality. Another example is seen when individuals who are asked to deal with too many stressful situations respond by saying, "I just can't think about that right now." In other words, the person is dealing with a smaller piece of the total reality.

There are many ways of accomplishing therapeutic partitioning. Any avenue by which a person perceives or processes information can potentially become broken off from others, including consciousness, memory, identity, and sensory functions. Because these divisions involve faculties of perception, it might be incorrectly

assumed that the personality of the patient is the object of partitioning. Rather the opposite is more often true. The collective
resources and skills of the patient are integrated and brought to
bear on one small aspect of the problem situation. Therefore, it is
the clinical problem, as defined by the patient that is the object of
partitioning. In the way that a person will not be ready to ingest an
entire cow during a single meal, the practitioner slices up the substance of the therapy so that noxious realities can be digested one
small piece at a time.

Symptom definition

The moment that something is defined it is no longer a fluid reality. It becomes a fragment broken off from all of its other potential
manifestations. When a symptomatic behavior is defined, it begins
to lose its pervasive, nonvolitional character. Delineating when the
behavior occurs, where it occurs, its intensity, duration, and other
details of its manifestation makes the behavior more predictable
and more amenable to control.

In this way, a simple assessment question, such as "Exactly when
does the problem occur?" becomes a seamless part of a larger clinical strategy. When working with a man who has some unnamed,
uncontrollable problem, it will be difficult, if not impossible, to
make progress. Once the problem is defined as "sexual relations,"
it becomes a smaller part of his total life situation. When further
delineated as "premature ejaculation," then the problem becomes
a still smaller part. The question one might then wonder is, "Can
this fragment be broken down any further?"

Erickson partitioned premature ejaculation one step further by
having a man with similar circumstances explain exactly how
many minutes he could engage in sex before ejaculating. This
divided up the process. Sex, as a whole, was no longer the problem. Instead it was a certain point during sex that was problematic. Erickson then dealt with the inevitability of the premature
ejaculation by suggesting that he experience "partial ejaculation"
at the appointed time and save the rest for a longer period of sex.
Thus, even the ejaculation itself was partitioned out. This was

something the man felt he could do and as a result his performance during sex improved substantially (Erickson, 1959d).

In some cases, the patient is overwhelmed by the feeling of never being free from the symptom, especially if it is pain or intense distress. Under these circumstances an innocuous question such as, "How often does the problem occur?" can provide surprising results. Sometimes there is an immediate change of facial expression as the patient starts to think about times when he or she is free of the symptom. This assessment question subtly begins the process of fragmenting the experience of symptomatic distress. This same technique has been thoroughly elaborated within the context of solution-focused therapy (de Shazer, 1994). Using this approach, the assessment is conducted as an intervention by identifying exceptions to the problem. The patient is then encouraged to elaborate on examples of when the problem behavior does not occur. The result is that the problem goes from being all-encompassing to something that represents only one portion of the patient's life experience.

The essence of what was to become solution-focused therapy was very nicely explained by Erickson during a 1962 lecture. While describing the significance of *how* you define the symptom, Erickson outlined the proper method for examining a sprained ankle. If it is the left ankle that is sprained, the practitioner should first ask to see the right ankle. He needs to examine this ankle in order to have a better understanding of what a normal ankle looks like on this individual. Then, when looking at the sprained ankle, the practitioner will be able to point out not only what is wrong with the sprained ankle but also what is right (Erickson, 1962a). This type of assessment not only helps break up the size of the problem but also provides some degree of hope.

Formal diagnosis

Case report: The woman who was mentally ill

A woman came to Erickson and said she was nervous. She complained, "The confounded neighbors, you know, even way at the end of the block, have such disagreeable voices. They are distressing me, disturbing my sleep and making me nervous." Her husband tried to argue with her. He wanted her to recognize that she could not hear the neighbors at the end of the street. But she insisted that she could hear them for at least two blocks around, even when they whispered. The more he tried to convince her otherwise, the more infuriated she became.

After listening to her story, Erickson told her that he thought she should go to the hospital, that she ought not to see him or any other psychiatrist on an outpatient basis. The woman responded by asking if Erickson thought she was crazy. Using a serious tone Erickson replied, "I would be ashamed to use that word crazy. I am a medical man. And I don't use that kind of language. But I do think you are mentally ill." He explained that he ought to tell her that just as he would tell her if she were physically ill. Erickson elaborated, "For physical illness you go to a hospital that takes care of physical illness. For the mental illness that you've got, you ought to go to a mental hospital."

While describing the outcome, Erickson reports, "The woman discussed it with me fairly intelligently but said she'd have to go home and talk it over. Her husband tried to argue with her that she really ought to see another psychiatrist and nobody would have such a gloomy view as I had." The woman said to her husband, "He was honest with me. He told me I was mentally ill. You've been telling me I can't hear somebody two blocks away. When I stopped to think about it, I never could, until I got this nervous and maybe that doctor is right." A couple days later, she insisted on being committed for hospital care as a mentally ill patient.

(Erickson, 1962a)

As a psychologist who formerly worked in the schools, Short has had the repeated experience of conducting the required assessment and, while sharing the diagnostic impressions with the student's parents, had a response such as, "It is a relief to finally know this." But why is it a relief? Why, in some instances, would parents show less distress after hearing that their son is autistic, than before they entered the office?

Diagnostic labeling has been attacked in the postmodernist literature as something that is overly reductionistic and dehumanizing.
There is the concern of stigmatizing the person with clinical labels.
However, this line of reasoning does not recognize the fact that
people who are not making social adjustments are *constantly* being
labeled by their failures and are frightened by the idea that they
are the *only* person to experience these difficulties. However, if it is
the *problem* that is appropriately labeled, rather than the *person*,
then a new entity is created—one that can be broken off from the
core of the individual identity. Once again, the problem is defined
in such a way that it is no longer a fluid reality.

Interestingly, positive results can also be achieved by administering a standardized test of psychopathology. In recent years
researchers have collected increasing amounts of data indicating
that significant relief from psychological and psychosomatic
symptoms can be achieved simply by administering the
Minnesota Multiphasic Personality Inventory and then sharing the
results in a feedback session (Finn and Tonsager, 1997).
Therapeutic benefit is derived seemingly without the use of any
formal therapeutic intervention. By sharing the results of this
inventory of psychopathology, the patients are given new perspectives as well as a vocabulary that effectively fragments their
perception of distress.

In many cases, when a formal diagnosis is provided, the patient
feels less overwhelmed and less confused because now the problems coming from the identified mental illness can be separated
from other problems of daily living. Before the partitioning was
orchestrated, the person was less able to allocate problem solving
energy to any one task because of an overly generalized idea that,
"I am a person who is not capable of dealing with life" or, in the
case cited above, "I am crazy." These stigmatizing thoughts encap-
sulate the entire identity leaving no resources for recovery.
However, after separating clinical from nonclinical concerns, the
individual is able to think, "So this is the disorder. Now what am
I going to do about it?" In the case example above, the woman was
completely overwhelmed by the voices of her neighbors. She was
enraged because she could not get her husband to believe her. But
Erickson was able to reduce the problem down to a single label

that had acceptable implications. When used respectfully, a formal diagnosis can give the patient direction, purpose, and hope.

Prognostic splitting

Case report: Cathy's cancer pain

Erickson was asked to see a woman suffering from extreme cancer pain. She had metastases in her lungs and in the bones of her thigh and pelvis. The intolerable pain had not been relieved by morphine, Demerol or any other narcotic. Erickson entered Cathy's room with her physician. She was chanting two urgent statements, "Don't hurt me. Don't scare me. Don't hurt me. Don't scare me. Don't hurt me …" Cathy was only 36 years old and had three children, the oldest was only eleven. She knew she had only a couple of months left to live.

Erickson immediately secured her attention: "But I must hurt you. I must scare you. I must hurt you. I must scare you. But just a little."

Next Erickson suggested Cathy remain awake from the neck up and that she let her body go to sleep. Using an urgent tone, he said, "I don't know why. I don't know what it means. But you must get an itch on the bottom of your foot." Cathy, who was in desperate need of relief from pain, resisted his suggestion: "I am sorry but I cannot develop an itch. All I can feel is numbness on the heel of my foot." Erickson expressed polite regret that she had not been able to develop an itch, and then suggested that the numbness gradually extend over her feet, legs, pelvis, and eventually to her neck. But, when it came to her chest, Erickson observed, "There is still an area of ulceration at the site of the surgery. I am sorry but I cannot remove this pain." Cathy acknowledged his regret and forgave him for his "failure." They both agreed that the remaining pain was a minor one and that she could cope with it. Erickson reports that he saw her on February 27 and that she remained mostly free of pain until she lapsed into a coma on August 25 followed by a rapid death.

(Erickson, 1962a)

As with all the strategies, partitioning should be understood within the context of providing aid to the patient rather than performing a "cure." This allows room for lack of perfection. Rather than having to resolve *all* aspects of a symptom complex, it may be that the patient is successful in doing away with 90 percent of the problem. Perhaps only the most troubling symptoms are alleviated. For those practitioners concerned by the idea of not "curing" patients, the question is asked, "Isn't an outcome of partial success more desirable than no progress at all?"

Healing is most likely to occur when there is a shift away from all-or-nothing thinking to thoughts about what can be accomplished. The introduction of this idea and collaborative review of possibilities is identified in this text as prognostic splitting. The objective is to *split the impossible from what is possible*. The effort is collaborative because ultimately it is the patient who decides what can be accomplished.

This same therapeutic strategy is used by many individuals seeking help from Alcoholics Anonymous. While developing the strength to battle a seemingly unyielding problem, the Serenity Prayer is invoked, "God grant me the serenity to accept the things I cannot change, the courage to change the things I can, and the wisdom to know the difference."[1] Such a self-assessment is, in fact, a prognostic splitting of situational factors.

Another common use of prognostic partitioning is accomplished by introducing the idea of stages. Thanks to the pioneering work of stage theorists such as Kübler-Ross (1969), individuals faced with death are not trapped by an indefinite period of isolation and denial. That is only the first stage and when recognized as such it becomes split off from the eventual outcome. The stages of anger, bargaining, and depression are also split off and the patient can look forward to the final stage of acceptance. In the way that a long-distance runner watches for the five-mile mark, and then the ten-mile mark, and so on, a patient who is experiencing suffering and pain will benefit from the ability to mark progress in relation to one piece of the overall problem. A common statement is, "The problem was too big for me to think about. I just needed to focus

---

[1] Reinhold Niebuhr, a prayer said to have been first published in 1951.

on some small area and see some progress." Another advantage of compartmentalizing a problem with stages is that it provides the patient with a map to the "final stage" in which the problem is resolved. With this new sense of direction comes hope.

This strategy is most effective when the patient is able to anticipate and recognize signs that identify each stage. The process of watching for signs and marking progress legitimizes the outcome predicted by the practitioner. While working with obstetrical patients, Erickson would acknowledge their need to experience some of the labor pain by describing the stages of birth and delivery. Erickson would explain that labor has three stages. He would then point out that they will be too busy during the second stage and third stage to pay full attention to the labor pain, so they should feel it during the first stage. He explained this technique, stating, "I have structured the situation so they can feel the contractions at a time when it will be less disturbing." In some cases, Erickson would describe labor as having five or six stages, especially if the woman seemed to need more than one stage during which to experience her contractions (Erickson, 1959a). For Erickson, it did not matter how many stages were used to fragment the problem: the more essential thing was to acknowledge the inevitability of discomfort as only one small part of the total outcome. As we all know, real life is never as tidy and perfectly sequenced as is a theoretical construct.

Another interesting version of prognostic splitting is achieved using the mind–body split. When working with individuals who suffered from some severe form of physical disability, Erickson would often preface his clinical work by stating, "There is an organic basis to your pain. And there is nothing I can do about that. However there is also a psychological component and that is something we can work on." After separating organic from the psychological aspects of a problem, the patient was able to take deliberate action in an area in which he or she can exercise some control. For example, while working with a boy who was suffering from asthma, Erickson explained, "Part of your asthma is organic and part is due to fear." Erickson then demonstrated how difficult it is to breath when a person becomes nervous and tightens the muscles in his chest. The knowledge that he could have some control over this part of his problem helped the boy to feel less frightened. As a result, the frequency and severity of his asthma attacks was reduced (Erickson, 1960c).

The most basic type of prognostic splitting is an essential element in any good treatment plan. When agreeing to therapy, each patient has a right to be informed of the known risks and benefits associated with treatment. If it is not likely that the patient will derive 100 percent improvement within the timeframe they desire, then some explanation should be made of what benefits the patient can expect and what constitutes a reasonable amount of time for them to occur. This procedure splits up rigid all-or-nothing thinking, while still providing hope.

While a treatment plan is being worked on, there should also be some discussion about the order of recovery. The patient is respectfully engaged in the process by asking him which symptoms he wants to address first and which symptoms he believes will be the first to relent. Some patients are able to be very precise in describing how they will respond to therapy and how long it will take to achieve their purposes; there are others who have absolutely no idea.

For individuals who cannot envision their own path to recovery, it can be helpful for the clinician to share some of his experiences with other people facing similar circumstances. In this way, a path to recovery is laid out. The patient starts to get an idea of how much relief he can expect and how long it will take. Although it is impossible for any practitioner have complete knowledge of future events, these prognostic estimates provide a structure on which hope is built.

In the case of Cathy's cancer pain, Erickson incorporated a very subtle and elegant form of partitioning. A prognostic split was made in relation to the amount of suffering she could expect to experience in the future. Before Erickson began therapy, pain was an experience that consumed all of Cathy's mind and body. In the end, the experience of pain was broken down and localized in only one part of her body, her ulcerated breast. The task of breaking her pain up into fragments began when Erickson suggested an itch on her foot, which would be adding a new piece of discomfort. The simple logic is if you can add a piece of pain, you can later take it away. Erickson explains, "My purpose in suggesting that was merely to start Cathy functioning within herself, to start her using her own body learnings and to use them according to her own pattern of response."

Not knowing how she would respond, Erickson then utilized her spontaneous development of numbness using the strategy of progression—taking something small and gradually increasing its size. He had the wisdom to recognize that Cathy's situation was not one that could be associated with pain-free living. Therefore, he gave her the option of retaining smaller fragments of her pain. This type of thinking made it possible for the most painful and troublesome symptoms to be overcome. When broken down in this way, even the most monumental of trials can be tolerated (Erickson-Klein, 1990, p. 280). Although this use of prognostic splitting was certainly not the only strategy employed, it provided an important opening for additional interventions.

Dividing the conscious from the unconscious

Case report: *The student's traumatic memory*

While teaching in medical school, Erickson was approached by a student who was curious about recovering a long-forgotten memory. Erickson agreed to use him as a demonstration subject. In a deep state of trance, the student announced, "I'm getting scared, awful scared, but I can't think of anything." Within a few minutes he developed a look of terror that seriously alarmed the students observing the demonstration.

Falteringly he gasped, "I'm scared, and I'm going to get sick. But I don't know why." The student began retching. His breathing became labored and spasmodic, his hands clasped and unclasped convulsively, and he seemed ready to collapse. Erickson introduced a series of breaks, during which he was brought out of trance, followed by more hypnotic work.

The student declared, "It's too big, I can't do it. Tell me how." Erickson responded, "You say it's too big. Why not do it a part here and a part there, instead of the whole thing at once, and then put the parts together into the whole big thing?"

Later the student was awakened with instructions to rest and to have a comprehensive amnesia for what had happened in the trance. He awakened, wiped the perspiration from his face and remarked that he must have eaten something that disagreed with him because he felt sick to his stomach. Later, after being returned to a hypnotic state, the student smiled and said, "That's funny. A scene just flashed into my mind. It's just as clear as if I were there. I'm back in Oklahoma. Let's see. I'm almost eight years old." He then experienced a final fit of terror as the full traumatic memory came to consciousness.

As a child he had been playing in the barn with a boy named Johnny. A fight developed and, while they were wrestling with a pitchfork, he stabbed Johnny in the leg. When Johnny screamed, he jerked the tine out and was horrified by the pulsing stream of blood. After calling a doctor, his father seized him and spanked him thoroughly, as he lay over his father's knees staring at the green scum of algae in the horse trough. His father then dragged him to the house and made him stand and watch while the doctor treated Johnny.

The doctor administered antitetanus serum, explaining the reason. Upon learning this, the father again beat his son. Just before the doctor left, Johnny developed anaphylactic shock. His eyes swelled shut, his tongue enlarged and protruded from his mouth, and he became a "horrible greenish color." He saw the doctor give another injection, insert a spoon into Johnny's mouth, and then take out a scalpel probably in preparation to give Johnny a tracheotomy. With only a child's understanding, the boy was all the more terrified that Johnny was to be "butchered like a pig."

All that night he dreamed of Johnny's skin turning a "horrible green like the horse trough." The next day he was forced to watch the doctor redress the wound, which was surrounded by "an awful color, green and nasty." Later that day, he neglected to pump water for the horses, and was again thoroughly spanked by his father, in the same position, and again looking into the scum of the horse trough.

After retrieving this memory, the student left class tired and exhausted. The other students were instructed not to discuss the matter. A week later the student visited Erickson, stating that he had learned some amazing things about himself as a result of his recovered memory. He was no longer as seriously interested in psychiatry. Instead he began a study of internal medicine. Secondly, his attitude toward dermatology had changed. Previously, he had been unable to study the textbook, despite repeated efforts. Each time he went to the dermatology clinic, he became sick and had to leave. Also, despite frequent faculty warnings, he had consistently avoided lectures given on the subject. Now he was studying dermatology with interest, and he enjoyed the clinics.

(Erickson, 1955/2001)

Although the use of partitioning, in one form or another, can be found in nearly every form of psychotherapy, the most dramatic examples can be found in hypnotherapeutic procedures. In hypnosis the most routine means of dividing awareness is to speak in terms of the conscious mind versus the unconscious. In fact, the fundamental concept of "going into a trance" suggests a partitioning of perception and information processing.

Erickson used hypnosis as one of his most versatile clinical tools. His trance inductions varied in style, formality, and duration; but each hypnotic induction brought about a separation of the conscious from the unconscious mind. Once a partitioning of conscious awareness was achieved, Erickson went on to guide the focus of attention toward a healing process.

For instance, while in trance the patient would be encouraged to use the "unconscious mind" to communicate an exceedingly painful idea, one that was previously too threatening to communicate or even consider. After the information was reviewed, Erickson would offer the patient the option of leaving it in the unconscious until he was ready to remember at the conscious level.

One of the greatest advantages of the Ericksonian hypnotic technique is that it helps patients learn to trust themselves. No matter how critical they may be of their thinking and judgment, the unconscious mind is always available as an untapped resource. As hypnotic phenomena are made manifest, such as an arm levitating automatically into the air, patients are encouraged to recognize the goodness of their own unconscious learnings and abilities. This resource, hidden outside the bounds of conscious awareness, gives patients the opportunity to view a piece of their mind as completely reliable. The clinical application of this concept promotes both an increase in self-efficacy and an internal locus of control, factors that are both associated with more favorable treatment outcomes.

Two well-known hypnotic techniques frequently used to facilitate fragmented conscious awareness are ideomotor signaling and automatic writing. Erickson (1961/2001b) developed these techniques following a series of discoveries that began with his experience in the rocking chair following the attack of polio (see p. xii). During the 1920s and 1930s, Erickson discovered automatic writing, hand levitation, and finally ideomotor signaling (Erickson, Rossi, and Rossi, 1976, p. 79). With ideomotor signaling a "yes" signal and a "no" signal are established by identifying specific movements in the head or fingers. Questions are then asked directly of the unconscious mind. This maneuver requires the subject's attention be distracted in one way or another so that the automatic movements are not observed. Thus subjects are asked to close their eyes or drift off into their own thoughts. To reduce the overall amount of self-consciousness, Erickson's preference was to ask for a subtle nonvolitional shaking or nodding of the head (*ibid.*). This is a behavior that often occurs automatically, regardless of whether or not a trance has been induced. The meaning of this automated action is reliable enough that it has been used with great success in the detection of lies (Ekman, 1992).

Automatic writing is a more complicated procedure in which a person is trained to move the fingers automatically with a pen or pencil in hand. Erickson was so skilled at this technique that he was able to achieve successful results even with individuals who were highly skeptical of their ability to write automatically (Erickson, 1958e). The outcome of automatic writing is a sort of doodling that produces words or sentences without requiring conscious attention. In some instances, it may be a series of pictures or symbols that is depicted (Erickson and Kubie, 1938/2001). As in ideomotor signaling, questions are asked that only a certain part of the mind can answer: "You can write that material without knowing what it is; then, you can go back and discover you know what it is without knowing you've done it" (Erickson, Rossi, and Rossi, 1976, p. 70). As has been discovered from research with brain-injured patients, the task of *writing* a response engages a different part of the brain than the task of typing a response or providing an oral reply (Carlson, 2004, p. 509). In this regard, the psychological strategy of partitioning highlights the presence of physiological boundaries in the constitution of the brain. By the soliciting of information from either a conscious or unconscious mind, the vastly complex processes of the brain are further stimulated.

Although the terms "conscious mind" and "unconscious mind" are not common in modern cognitive research, a nearly identical concept has been delineated using the terms "implicit" and "explicit" memory. These terms are also synonymous with "declarative" and "nondeclarative" memories. Put simply, explicit (or declarative) memory is any memory of events that can be talked about or examined with logic. It contains all of the concrete details associated with the recalled information. In contrast, implicit (or nondeclarative) memory is the recall of information that includes instances of perceptual, stimulus–response, and/or motor learning, which exist without awareness. These memories operate automatically, controlling behavior without the benefit of reason. With this type of recall the individuals do not have access to the facts or experiences that have led to their responses. Similarly, an implicit memory can trigger a strong emotional reaction without any cognizance of a specific event to which the feelings belong. This duality, described by Erickson as the conscious versus the unconscious mind, reflects the biological partitions of the mind. Research has shown that explicit memories are dependent on the hippocampal formation, while implicit memories are not (Carlson, 2004). The fact that different portions of the brain process information in different ways is a biological reality that should be recognized and employed in a strategic rather than random fashion. As was demonstrated in the previous case report, the practitioner merely needs to offer the opportunity of processing information separately.

During his work with the medical student, Erickson commented on how the traumatic memory might be recovered. He guided the process by asking the following questions: Did the student want the whole thing to erupt into his conscious mind all at once? Or would he prefer to have it come piecemeal, one part at a time, with the possibility of halting the process and mustering his strength so that he could more easily endure the next development? Would he want to separate the affective from the cognitive elements and experience the one or the other first? Or would he like to have the recovery follow the same course of development, the same chronology, as the original experience? (Erickson, 1955/2001.) As this case demonstrates, when an overwhelming reality is broken apart in various ways, the traumatic memory can be more easily assimilated. It is also important to note that this review was conducted within the context of a safe environment. Although recent research findings challenge the accuracy of hypnotically retrieved memories, for the purposes of this discussion it is safe to say that the reprocessing of information, facilitated by Erickson, was meaningful to the patient.

This methodology is not only useful for processing traumatic memories but might also be employed while dealing with the patient's fear of change. Individuals who are afraid to marry, to have children, or otherwise change their life conditions might be assisted by discussing these possibilities only during trance while using the unconscious mind. After the person comes out of trance, these threatening ideas are fragmented from "normal consciousness" by giving the person permission to develop a hypnotic amnesia for discussions that occurred during trance. A common maxim of Erickson's was, "Consciously remember what you want to remember but remember some things can be left in your unconsciousness where they can *really* help you." The point here is not an argument for or against the reality of the trance state or the reality of the unconscious mind. The important thing to recognize is the ease by which partitioning can be achieved, and the benefits that develop as a result.

Dissection

While most clinicians are familiar with the term "Oriented × 3," not many would admit to intentional manipulation of the patient's orientation to person, place, or time by means of partitioning. Yet this is a common practice. When a patient comes to the psychoanalyst and discovers that his once total personality is now a combination of the id, ego, and superego, he is going to experience a new orientation to person. When the patient comes to see the clinician who is trained in transactional analysis, then he is likely to leave the session more keenly aware of his domineering parent ego state and all the trouble that can now be attributed to it. Any mapping out of psychodynamics requires partitioning psychological realities and, as many different schools of psychotherapy have discovered, it generally aids the patient in the process of creating goals and identifying targets for change.

Using learning theory as the philosophical base, behavior analysts have developed a systematic means of dissecting behavior using a technique called "functional analysis." This use of partitioning provides a logical framework in which to understand behavioral patterns. Functional analysis is intended to draw attention to environmental factors that contribute to the maintenance of problem behavior. The dissection of behavior is accomplished by identifying three components: the *antecedent*, the *discrete behavior*, and the *consequence*. This is also known as the ABC theory (Shapiro and Kratochwill, 1988). In order to modify the behavior (B), the clinician can attempt to alter the antecedents (A), the consequences (C), or both. For example, Short recently witnessed a mother who was struggling with her son's tantrums. During their time at the park, she often made requests of the child that she was not entirely willing to enforce. "Johnny, we are going home. No more playing at the park." This was followed by a predictable, discrete behavior. Johnny fell to the ground and began to scream and flail. His mother was overwhelmed and told Johnny that if he would stop screaming he could play fifteen more minutes on the playground. As a consequence for throwing tantrums, he was rewarded with more of whatever he wanted. As a result of the embarrassing tantrums, one might imagine his mother felt even more reluctant to assert her wishes in the future, which then becomes the antecedent for the next occurrence of tantruming. It is only after the behavior is dissected in this way that a means of escape from this self-perpetuating spiral becomes apparent. Although it might seem somewhat mechanical, the usefulness of this form of dissection is not to be underestimated. As argued by Michael Yapko (2003), a leading scholar on Ericksonian therapy, "… you must understand a symptom's function(s) and provide alternatives that satisfy the symptom's underlying need without having to have the destructive symptom present" (p. 408).

The most dramatic examples of dissection can be found in experiential therapies such as Gestalt therapy, psychodrama, and in hypnosis. When a patient is asked to look at an empty chair and then talk to her mother, a most definite division takes place as the person dissociates from the day-to-day experience of self-identity. Similarly, while constructing a drama, a patient might be asked to role-play himself at different time periods in his lifetime. This partitioning creates new options as one aspect of the identity is pitted against the other. Each of these techniques might simultaneously alter all three spheres of general reality orientation, within the context of a controlled therapeutic exercise.

In the way that a person can be dissected along theoretical psychodynamics, it is also possible to work on smaller pieces of the total identity by examining parts of the body. When working with individuals who had a disturbed body image or who were afraid of biological functions such as sex, Erickson would often employ a technique he referred to as "microcosmic self-examination." For instance, while working with a woman who complained of frigidity, Erickson pulled out his medical textbooks and helped her study each fiber and tissue of the female reproductive system. After considering each of these small pieces of her anatomy, and after discussing the individual functions of each organ and piece of tissue, Erickson turned to the topic of orgasm. He asked her how much use her hand would be if she could feel only one side of it. She agreed that her hand should have feeling on both sides. Therefore, Erickson encouraged her to experiment with feeling her orgasm on the left side of the labia on one occasion of intercourse and then on the right side of the labia during a different occasion. This way she did not have to assimilate the experience of orgasm all in one large chunk but instead in parts, spread out across time. Following this meeting, the woman reported that she was now capable of very satisfying orgasms (Erickson, 1960b). This partitioning and microcosmic examination of her physical anatomy reduced the emotional power of the negative thoughts associated with sex and helped her develop a new understanding of herself and her sexuality.

Partitioning of time and space

Case report: The man who could not drive out of town

> A man who was experiencing intense panic attacks came to Erickson for help. He was able to leave his house but could drive only down certain streets. His phobic avoidances were continuing to increase as his ability to move about was steadily decreasing. Most of all, he was certain that he could not drive past the city limits without fainting behind the wheel of his car. Understanding these conditions, Erickson instructed the man to take his car out into the desert, on a deserted street, late in the night. At the city limit, he was to pull his car over and lie in the ditch next to the road. After a prescribed amount of time, he was to get back into his car, drive to the next telephone pole, stop and again lie in the ditch. The man was told to wear one of his nice suits and was provided with a doctor's note that would be pinned to the lapel, in case he was discovered by the police. He did as he was instructed. After a while he grew tired of the ordeal, so he drove his car in a regular unrestricted fashion to the next town.

> (Erickson, 1958f)

A trend in modern forms of therapy is to reject the idea that assessment and intervention must exist as two mutually exclusive events. Methods of assessment used in behavioral therapies and postmodern therapies are most often viewed as the beginning of intervention. A clear understanding of partitioning makes this point even more obvious. With questions such as, "When is your problem felt most intensely?" and "Where are you when the problem usually occurs?" the process of assessment simultaneously acts as a therapeutic agent by breaking apart the size of the problem. Rather than being overwhelmed by the problem at all moments, the patient can recognize significant exceptions.

For example, Short interviewed a small boy whose face was contorted in pain. "I just can't take it any more! I just can't take all of this stress!" he said. After Short asked him to describe which circumstances were most likely to cause him stress, there was immediate evidence of lessened tension in his face and shoulders. The events that really bothered him occurred only two or three times a week. This did not resolve all of the boy's problems but the burden no longer felt so large.

Other examples of this widely used strategy can be found outside the context of traditional therapy. Dale Carnegie recognized the value of partitioning by instructing those who struggle with worry to break their tasks up into "day-tight compartments." Alcoholics Anonymous has incorporated the same strategy by creating the mantra, "one day at a time." This single strategy has proved itself to be a major turning point in the lives of many an individual.

When working with physical pain as the symptom, Erickson found it useful to fragment the pain by discussing the difference between immediate, remembered, and anticipated experience (Erickson, 1959b). He would treat these as equal intervals and then suggest amnesia for the remembered pain and amnesia for the future pain, thereby eliminating "two-thirds" of the problem (Erickson, 1958c). Of course, the exact amount of pain reduction that is to be accomplished is not as important as the hope that *some* reduction in pain will occur.

This technique is most effective when the pain is cyclic. In one such case, a man was dying of cancer. His suffering was intolerable and came in the form of sharp lancinating pain every ten minutes followed by dull heavy aching pain. When the lancinating pain came the man cried out in an uncontrollable fashion. Erickson employed a number of procedures, such as hypnotic dissociation and distraction, "You can enjoy watching that young nurse over there" (a hallucinated nurse). However his primary intervention was to break up the man's pain across time. Erickson explained to him that his memory of the pain was one-third of his pain. Anticipating the next occurrence of pain was another third. The third and final portion was the actual duration of the acute pain experience. Because narcotics had not been effective in abolishing the pain, Erickson told him it was asking a bit too much to expect hypnosis to abolish all of the pain. So the pain was reduced to one-third of its original size. The man still cried out in pain every so often, but he did not remember the experience of the pain, nor did he anticipate any future pain (Erickson, 1959b). This method lends itself well to work with pain because the worst type of pain is that which is unending. When time is compartmentalized, resiliency is increased; and if the pain does not seem that it will be unending, then hope is produced as well.

When partitioning a person's reality orientation, Erickson would often work in three domains—person, place, and time—simultaneously. In the case of Rebecca and her reaction to repeated attacks from a vicious dog (see p. 15); partitioning played a central role in the healing process. When commenting on this case, Erickson pointed out that, as often happens with traumatized individuals, Rebecca's need to avoid harm became overgeneralised and resulted in an intense fear of leaving the security of her house. Erickson began therapy by providing her with a good view of herself. He helped her laugh and feel unafraid.

Time was then fragmented by his pointing out the difference between how awful and fearful she felt after the attack versus her feelings at the current moment. He then began the task of fragmenting space by pointing out that at the current location she was happy and if she was at the property of the dog she would be frightened. Similarly, she could be at any number of places and not be frightened, as long as the dog was not there. This she could agree to.

Erickson then partitioned off the entity of the dog by describing his own harmless basset. After she met and enjoyed petting Erickson's gentle dog, he pointed out that it was not every dog that frightened her. It was the great big aggressive dogs that frightened her. All of these statements were agreeable to Rebecca and therefore acceptable as a new reality orientation (Erickson, 1963).

The case at the beginning of the section, the man fearful of driving, illustrates Erickson's use of space as a means of fragmenting a problem that previously seemed insurmountable. It was the reality of unlimited space that was most overwhelming. So Erickson used telephone poles to create compartments outside the boundary of the city limits. After making it successfully from one telephone pole to another, the man was able to recognize that he could travel from city to city, which was simply a generalization of the strategy introduced by Erickson. A point that should not be missed, is that he was "all dressed up with no place to go," so he drove to Flagstaff. Unfortunately, we do not have any further information on what he did once he arrived.

The general application of partitioning

As mentioned throughout this chapter, partitioning is not a specific technique but instead a strategy that underlies the form and function of a general approach to healing. Techniques are narrowly defined behavioral protocols that have limited application. Each technique works best with certain problems and certain personality types. However, strategies such as partitioning provide principles from which clinical judgment is derived and from which interventions are produced.

The logic of partitioning applies to any effort to recognize resources existing within patients. In other words, if the person cannot cope with the entirety of this situation, then what small part are they ready to take on? A similar question dictated by this type of logic might be, "When, where, and how will the person feel more capable of dealing with the problem?" This is the type of internal dialogue that was undoubtedly a part of Erickson's implicit reasoning. This logical framework prepares the practitioner to identify resources in the patient and fosters a readiness to deal with distressing variables one after another rather than trying to tackle the complete problem all at once.

As with all of the clinical strategies described in this book, partitioning can be misused by the practitioner and possibly damage therapeutic relationships. The primary contraindication for this strategy is any case in which the patient would feel that his or her concerns are not being taken seriously. It is possible to minimize unintentionally the patient's suffering by not respecting the patient's right, or even desire, to experience suffering. This is especially likely to happen when the practitioner is uncomfortable witnessing suffering and is tempted to respond with messages such as, "It's really not that bad" or "You'd feel a lot better if you just looked at things differently." This is not a true form of partitioning. Any effort to minimize the legitimacy of the patient's suffering is rude, dismissive, and likely to encourage resentment. Even hopeful statements, such as, "The prognosis is good" can have this unintended effect, if the patient's perspective is not taken into account. Whenever a patient told Erickson about how sad and miserable he was, Erickson was careful to acknowledge the statement and accept it as fact. Erickson knew it was only after the patient had his or her reality respected, that progress could be made toward new, equally acceptable ideas. For example, "It hurts awful bad right now. And it will probably keep on hurting for a little while." This was a message from Erickson to his three-year-old son Robert after he had fallen down the stairs and knocked his tooth up into the maxilla (Erickson, 1958/2001). Erickson's statement fragmented time. Instead of a lifetime of suffering, with the words "probably" and "a little while" he provided his son with the hope and the idea that the pain would not last much longer. His statement was truthful yet neither dismissive nor insulting.

Chapter 9

Progression

This chapter describes the strategy of progression and its function in therapy. This strategy provides a basic context in which all other problem solving strategies are implemented. The five techniques listed here provide a small sample of the numerous ways in which therapeutic progression can be achieved. The chapter begins with a case example that Erickson used to explain the concept of progression. As will be seen, all great journeys begin with one small step.

Case report: The man who cursed life

As described earlier (see p. 7), a man was brought to Erickson after spending eleven years sitting in wheelchair due to extremely painful arthritis. He was in such poor condition that he could not move his knees, arms or much of his body and was capable only of a little movement in his thumb and neck. He spent his time uttering obscenities and feeling angry about his pitiful state. After meeting with Erickson over a period of months, he regained the ability to walk with the exception of a small limp and occasional periods of extended bed rest. While explaining this man's healing process Erickson commented, "My feeling was that, if he could move the distal joint of the thumb, then he could move the joint connected to it, and if he could move that, then he could move the next finger which was also connected, and then build up little by little more movement." Erickson's task was to motivate the man into some type of action for the purposes of healing. The therapeutic nature of this elicited action was the slow, incremental extension of his existing abilities. While admitting to his own limited knowledge of the future, Erickson confessed, "I didn't have any idea that a year later he would be out of the wheelchair and driving a truck. But he took all of that energy that he had been wasting on profanity and put it into the exercise of his thumb, fingers, arms, and eventually his body movement."

(Erickson, 1957)

"The beginning is the most important part of the work."
– Plato, c. 428–348 BCE

Progress is not likely when the clinical objective seems out of reach. In some cases, patients may find themselves so firmly entrenched in the expectation of inevitable failure that therapeutic maneuvers are ignored or passively resisted. Negative expectations can be difficult to overcome because of the patient's experiential understanding of the severity of the symptomatic behavior and a history of repeated failure. But, no matter how damaged a person may be, everyone has a point at which the therapeutic task is so small and so simple that he or she will give it a try. Like a brick stairway, most psychological resources can be built slowly and subtly, laying one brick on top of another, thereby creating a progression of meaningful steps. With each new sign of progress, the individual becomes stronger and more ready to meet the next challenge. Eventually the distance is eliminated between the low point at which the patient began and the pinnacle of the therapeutic objective. The same concept is reflected in the well-known saying, "Just take one small step at a time." Within the context of clinical problem solving, the practitioner is able to build seemingly impossible accomplishments on top of many smaller and simpler tasks.

A basic premise in Erickson's approach to therapy was that therapeutic change involves the introduction of immediate success experiences that are designed to persist and flourish far into the future (Robles, 1990). He approached clinical problems with a focus on both the here and now and the future. It is progression that provides the bridge between these two orientations so that both function in service to one another. Progression incorporates time as a functional component through which all other problem solving strategies are implemented.

Simply put, progression allows the practitioner to build on a series of small gains, creating increased hope for continued accomplishments. This therapeutic process is in some ways synonymous with the more commonly known concept of adaptation, which also involves a series of small cumulative changes. As the study of nature has shown, all creatures need time to adapt to changes in the environment. An even more gradual progression can be seen as all of nature slowly evolves over time. Accordingly, it is the gradual progression of events that results in sustainable change. The logical necessity of this is apparent when considering the example of a man who came to visit Erickson. He walked into the office and said, "I weigh 300 pounds. I want to leave here weighing 150 pounds." Erickson's question was, "When do you want to walk out of here weighing 150 pounds?" He repeated his demand, and added, "Today" (Erickson, 1962c). The man was not willing to invest any time in the process of recovery. He could not see the absurdity of his request.

Within the context of organic disease, we find that each person has his or her own pace at which progress is achieved. Some individuals recover quickly and some require greater amounts of time. Within the context of mental healing, this progression is usually linked to the development of new skills and the generation of hope. While conducting therapy it is essential that the patient recognize that a reasonable amount of time should be involved in recovery. Erickson (1958b) illustrated this concept with the following dialogue:

Patient: "How long will it take to cure my problem?"

Erickson: "Well, how long have you had your problem?"

Patient: "Ten years."

Erickson: "Well, I certainly do not want to take as long to cure you as it took for you to develop your problem and to bring it in to me. It ought to be done in a much shorter time than ten years. But let's be reasonable about it. Give me a reasonable length of time."

Both the patient and the practitioner need realistic expectations that are linked to some form of progression. Rather than hoping for an instant cure, there is a vigilant watch for some evidence of progress, thereby creating an ever increasing expectation of success.

Within the context of trauma work, it is especially important to recognize the patient's fear of failure. Dolan (2000) believes that reluctant behaviors commonly interpreted as resistance, or low motivation, are actually fear of failure. Yapko (2003) makes a similar point when he describes resistance as a form of communication. This type of behavior reveals the patient's most deeply felt limitations. Dolan's approach to this issue, especially at the beginning of therapy, is to have patients identify and focus on steps that are so small that the patient begins to feel a little impatient. This is the beginning of a forward momentum that progresses once it is reinforced and capitalized upon. Dolan (2000) emphasizes the importance of focusing on *very small steps*. As a rule, the more traumatized people are, the more gentle the therapist must be when inviting them to self-disclose or to risk untested behaviors. Because the steps are extremely small, the patient has less risk of failing.

The statement, "Time heals all wounds," is not always true. However, it is true that all wounds require some amount of time to heal. And, in the way that a disease may progress over time, healing can have a gradual beginning and then progress into something further reaching in scope. Similarly, changes in behavior require learning, and learning takes time. Each new skill that is developed becomes the base for a new more sophisticated form of behavior. First, the changes are microscopic, then, like a funnel, they gradually broaden in scope. The strategy of progression can be recognized as a key component in almost all forms of sustainable change; however, the subtle beginnings of this process can be easily missed. In the way that one recognizes the progression of disease, clinicians must recognize and appreciate the progression of healing.

Progression is a crucial strategy for the effective handling of fear. In therapy, the patient must prepare for change and for dealing with the unknown. Both are frightening psychological factors that must be taken into account. When describing his efforts to pace therapy and not move too quickly, Erickson remarked, "… if I do it any faster, I will scare the daylights out of him. I will not get any results. I will terrify him. I will lose the patient. I will not do him one bit of good by saving time" (Erickson, 1962c). As explained by Erickson, time is something used by the practitioner to achieve certain results. Progression requires a willingness to spend time with the patient, to answer questions, listen to concerns, and reduce fears through gradual exposure.

Progression does not always have to be seen as a process of building something up. The strategy is also useful in bringing something down, such as the diminution of pain. Initially, the patient may be introduced to the idea that over the course of the next hour his pain can be diminished at some imperceptible level, perhaps only 0.005 percent. Once this idea is accepted, the momentum continues by diminishing the pain still further and further. Over a long period of time it gradually fades away (Erickson-Klein, 1990, p. 277). The patient has a lifetime of experiences indicating that this is in fact the way things work. But it is the introduction of hope that speeds up the process and greatly increases the patient's resiliency to ongoing experiences of discomfort.

When describing this strategy, Erickson often used the medical analogy of the method in which a physician feels for a swollen organ. The physician does not push down right in the center of the painful area. Instead he starts at the periphery and gently moves his fingers toward the hurt (Erickson, 1963). As can be said with all of the techniques of progression listed below, it is generally a good idea to start with an easy problem, some area where the patient is confident that progress can be made. Like the physician examining a swollen organ, the practitioner should start on a more peripheral issue and work in toward areas of greater pain and sensitivity.

Although many types of psychotherapy use progression, it is built into the very fabric of hypnosis and hypnotic induction in particular. Rather than be expected to instantly attain a state of hypnotic responsiveness, the subject is slowly guided into trance by means of progressive relaxation, or images of floating up, up, up to a cloud, or slowly levitating an arm one inch at a time, etc. These diverse techniques all have in common the element of gradual progression. In fact, trance deepening is almost always done as a series of small steps: "As I count from one to twenty, you will go deeper and deeper into trance… Each new time you go into trance, you will become more able to respond to suggestion… With every new breath, you are feeling more and more at ease." When used in hypnosis, progression becomes a microcosm for continued progress in therapy. The question, "Will I be able to go into trance?" anticipates the larger and more pervasive question, "Will therapy help me recover?" If the answer to the first question is yes, then the first small step toward healing has been achieved.

Psychotherapy as a whole is a progressive process. While discussing the importance of eliciting the patient's participation and cooperation, Erickson would often say, "If you can get them to move an inch, then you can topple them over." Change requires time and a readiness to participate. This concept is similar to the statement, "Every thousand-mile journey begins with one small step." In mental healing, the patient is generally encouraged to take one small step in the direction of what he or she recognizes as success. This gradual progress allows the patient time to develop the neurological, biological, and social structures necessary to sustain change.

Geometric progression

Case report: A case of intractable neurodermatitis

A man came to Erickson for help with intractable neurodermatitis. The rashy skin condition covered his body and caused him great discomfort. He suffered from insomnia and painful itching on his face, legs, arms, and back. After examining him, Erickson asked, "Would you be willing to improve unnoticeably?" Erickson explained that if he improved one-millionth of one percent in one week's time, and doubled the progress to two millionths of one percent in two weeks' time, and then four millionths of one percent after three weeks, that the change would most definitely remain unnoticeable. The man was immediately engrossed in the idea. Erickson pointed out that in 21 weeks he could improve one full percentage point and that still would be unnoticeable. However, he warned, "Eight more weeks of doubling the progress would bring it to 128 percent, which is too fast for the abatement of a life-long condition." The man agreed that was too fast and continued to follow with great interest the logic behind Erickson's insistence that progress remain slow.

This first visit was on March 17. His next appointment was set for four weeks, at which time he informed Erickson that he knew he was improving but it was absolutely unnoticeable. His third visit was mid-May and he made similar comments. On May 31 Erickson got an emergency call. It was the man and he explained, "While shaving, I suddenly noticed my face was not bleeding like it usually does. Then I realized that it had not been bleeding all week, like it usually does. And that surprised me. Then I happened to look at my chest and noticed that my clawing marks were missing and that my skin had practically healed up! I looked at my legs and they were better. Then I realized I had been sleeping every night for the past week, without any insomnia! I dressed and ran to tell my wife that my skin had improved and she agreed that it had. Then I suddenly remembered that I had taken my wife out to dinner twice that week. I have not done that for years and years. When I mentioned this to my wife she said she had felt that going out to eat was special but she did not want to mention it because she did not want to break her luck."

After this breakthrough, Erickson continued to monitor the man's progress. The patient's skin continued to improve. Additionally, he began taking up new hobbies such as reading. He began taking his wife out to dinner and on weekend trips. As a result the marriage became much happier.

(Erickson, 1960c)

> "If the camel once gets his nose in the tent,
> his body will soon follow."
> – Saudi Arabian proverb

While describing the strategy of progression, Erickson most frequently referenced a technique he called "geometrical progression." The procedure begins by introducing some small step toward future success, one that is so ridiculously small that it cannot be rejected. For example, Erickson might ask an insomniac to consider the possibility of adding just two minutes more sleep to one week's cumulative sleep. How can a person reject the possibility of perhaps accidentally sleeping two more minutes this week than the week before? The next step in the procedure is to introduce the idea of doubling gains. Erickson often asked his patients, "How much money would you have in only one month if you started with a penny and doubled the amount each day?"

Most people are shocked to learn that it amounts to more than $5 million. Geometrical progression is a concept of reality that communicates the idea that small, simple steps can eventually be of great value. For Erickson, this was used as a tool to help the patient make that first crucial step toward progress.

As defined above, progression is the process of gradually and systematically increasing the amount or frequency of desired behavior. It works best when the process begins slowly and with some infinitesimal step. Research shows that the rationales accompanying treatments should not promise too great an initial change (Kirsch, 1990). It is more important to get the patient to accept the idea that some degree of change can be achieved, so that small fluctuations in the problem condition can be interpreted as evidence of improvement (p. 51).

Geometrical progression is a cognitive technique designed by Erickson to justify the patient's initial investment of energy into the healing process. The technique helps create positive expectations for what eventually can be achieved using a modest beginning. Impact can be added to the technique by placing a penny in the person's hands and asking him or her to speculate on how many pennies there will be if the first penny is doubled on the first day, then the two pennies are doubled on the second day and that doubling of pennies is continued for a month. The answer is, more than 500 million pennies. Although not all individuals are excited by picturing large amounts of money, for many it is an engaging technique.

In the case above, the man probably felt self-conscious about his skin and desperate to have a condition that covered his entire body become less noticeable. Remember, he is an adult who has been told by a physician that he has *intractable* neurodermatitis, therefore his thinking processes are going to be oriented toward "covering it up" rather than the more hopeful idea that it can be healed. Erickson met the man's need to have his condition escape detection by offering progress that would be *unnoticeable*. Erickson explained it is often difficult to get the patient to accept improvement without constantly scrutinizing it (which only leads to more neurotic self-consciousness and increased psychosomatic symptomology). Erickson used geometric progression to turn this neurotic pattern on its tail by distracting the man with the happy expectation of a lack of noticeable progress.

Progressive desensitization

Case report: The woman who was slapped by her dentist

Jackie, a 21-year-old woman, walked cautiously into the office of a dentist and said, "I want to see you in your office. I do not want to talk with you where you have your dental chair." The dentist had been trained in hypnosis by Erickson. He said, "All right. Can you tell me why?" She said, "The last time I went to see a dentist was when I was a little girl. And he slapped my face until I stopped crying. Now I need some dental care and I am scared. I am awfully scared and I need some dental care. I would like to have you look at my mouth and tell me how much I need but please don't slap my face!" Jackie had neither brushed her teeth nor visited a dentist since the age of eight.

The dentist welcomed Jackie into his office and had her sit in a chair by the door. "Suppose you lean back in your chair and I will lean back in my chair, on the far side of this desk." Because she was visibly tense he said, "You seem awfully afraid of me. Aren't you glad that there is all of this distance between us?" After she had time to relax he pointed out that she could look down the hallway and see the dental chair but that she was closer to the exit than she was to the dental chair so she could just look at it without fear. The dentist let her know that this was enough work for one day, "And when do you think you would like to schedule your appointment? Don't schedule it too soon but take as long as you want to." She asked, "Would it be all right if I put it off until tomorrow?" He acknowledged her desire to put it off and respected this need by putting it off even more, "Well, let's make it late tomorrow."

When Jackie arrived for her appointment she was given the opportunity to sit in the dental chair without anyone else in the room. The dentist had told her to get comfortable, try out the cushion in the seat, and just look around the room. After having time to get comfortable she said that she would like to make an appointment for extractions but the dentist said, "Before making any extractions,

I would like to look into your mouth and you can hold it as wide open as you want to but not one bit wider than you want." She smiled and slowly opened her mouth, wider and wider. The dentist merely looked, without making any movements toward her face. Then he told her to close her mouth. All of her teeth were horribly decayed.

The dentist explained to Jackie that she would need dentures. Before scheduling the procedure he said, "I am going to touch your cheek and then your chin. I just want you to get acquainted with the feeling of my hand on your cheek and on your chin because when I do the extractions I am going to touch your face."

Eventually the extractions were completed. There was no complication. After this she was sent to a second dentist for the fitting of dentures and that went smoothly as well. Erickson, who had already worked with Jackie's sister, then met with her to help with future adjustments to college, dating, and her eventual marriage. The girl graduated from college and became a dental hygienist

(Erickson, 1963; Erickson, 1958a).

The strategy of progression is the central dynamic in many highly effective techniques. This is especially true of the hypnotic technique known as "progressive relaxation." The patient does not experience relief immediately or throughout the entire body. The relaxation begins in some small distant part, such as a toe, and then slowly moves to the toe next to it, and then the knee, and the hips, and the shoulders, etc. This process of progressive relaxation does not produce an instant cure but instead acts as a first step, the beginning of a larger progression of steps toward overcoming anxiety, or stress, or high blood pressure, etc. Progressive relaxation is often used in combination with gradual exposure to noxious stimuli resulting in what Wolpe (1969) initially termed "systematic desensitization." As with all forms of progression, therapeutic benefit is derived from the patient's exposure to something threatening but within the context of a safe environment.

During the heyday of psychoanalysis, the most widely used tool in psychotherapy was emotional catharsis. The principle of emotional catharsis was compared to the technology of the steam engine. In order to avoid breakdown, the engine had to have a method of releasing pressure. Similarly, Freud believed that instances of forgotten memory (traumata) must be recalled by some means (catharsis) in order to avoid an abnormal use of undischarged sums of excitement (conversion) (Freud, 1912/1966, p. 934). This single technique was so central to the development of psychotherapy that many professionals still treat the two terms (catharsis and psychotherapy) as synonymous.

Whenever this technique was employed by Erickson, it was done in a slow, permissive manner. He never rushed his patients but instead allowed them to move in the direction of catharsis using small fragmented steps or symbolic gestures. While explaining his use of catharsis Erickson stated, "A need in human living is to reexperience painful things within the context of a safe environment" (Erickson, 1964b). Thus therapeutic catharsis can be evaluated from the perspective of progressive desensitization. If a person can bring a painful event to consciousness, it loses a little bit of its power. When a person can then think about the event using different frames of reference, it again loses power. If the person can then talk about the event, it loses still more power. Finally, if the person can go through the visceral processes of reexperiencing the event, as often happens in hypnosis, then progression toward assimilation is complete. This process was illustrated well in the case of the student with the traumatic memory (see p. 67). The memory of having stabbed another boy with a pitchfork, watching him nearly die, and then the unrelenting corporal punishment by his father was too overwhelming. Fortunately, Erickson recognized his emotional needs and provided a safe environment and a slow progressive means of reexperiencing the event.

In addition to dealing with events from the past, progressive desensitization provides a useful means of dealing with immediate fears and self-imposed limitations. It is something that almost every child does naturally at about twelve months of age. In an unfamiliar environment, the cautious toddler moves only three or four feet from the safety of her mother's legs. Then she waits to see if she is safe. If she knows that her mother is watching, and the toddler can sense that Mom is not concerned about any of the events occurring around her, then she will move out another ten or so feet. After a moment of play, she might momentarily return to her mother, for a check in, but then she will be ready to go back out and explore yet further.

A wild animal, such as a squirrel, might do the same while trying to decide whether or not to go all the way up to a person's hand and take the food that is being offered. Erickson used a similar approach in what he described as one of his first experiments with a psychotherapeutic strategy:

> A patient in Worcester State Hospital, in Massachusetts, demanded he be locked in his room, where he spent his time anxiously and fearfully winding string around the bars of the window of the room. He knew his enemies were going to come in and kill him, and the window was the only opening. The thick iron bars seemed to him to be too weak, so he reinforced them with string. I went into the room and helped him reinforce the iron bars with string. In doing so, I discovered that there were cracks in the floor and suggested that those cracks ought to be stuffed with newspaper so that there was no possibility of his enemies getting him. Then I discovered cracks around the door that should be stuffed with newspaper. Gradually I got him to realize that the room was only one of a number of rooms on the ward, and to accept the attendants as a part of his defense against his enemies; and then the hospital itself as a part of his defense against his enemies; and then the Board of Mental Health of Massachusetts as part, and then the police system—the governor. Then I spread it to adjoining states. Finally I made the United States a part of his defense system. This enabled him to dispense with the locked door because he had so many other lines of defense.
>
> (Erickson and Zeig, 1977/2001, p. 1)

Although this intervention sounds as though it occurred during a single moment in time, Erickson undoubtedly spent a lot of time with this patient with each step of progression being accepted and then built upon. Rather than just talking about the possibility of movement and then leaving the patient out on his own, it is a safe guess that Erickson walked around the ward with the patient, helping him expand his zone of comfort. In response to this intervention, the patient was able to receive ground privileges and to move freely about the grounds. He ceased his frantic endeavors to protect himself and began productive work in the hospital shops (*ibid.*).

In the earlier case report, 'The woman who was slapped by her dentist,' the woman's movement across space and time, toward the dental chair, is the initial progressive technique. She was literally allowed to take one step at a time and to delay the procedure. This is a particularly straightforward illustration of progression, which reminds most of us what we as children learned about wild animals. They must always be approached in a slow manner, gradually allowing them to build a sense of security; otherwise they will just run away. This woman who needed dental work was extremely frightened. What the dentist provided was a slow progression toward the thing that she most feared within the context of a safe environment.

Pattern interruption

Case report: The man who had to urinate through a tube

During the World War II draft, a man who wanted to enter the military revealed a very embarrassing problem to Erickson, who was serving on the board of examiners. The man was unable to urinate unless he held an eight- to ten-inch pipe to the head of his penis. Erickson conducted a full psychiatric examination and decided that the man was reasonably well adjusted at work and in social regards. His problem with urination seemed to be linked to a childhood trauma.

As a small boy he had urinated through a knothole in a wooden fence by a golf course. Unfortunately he was apprehended in the act, severely punished, and humiliated. Having been unable to finish the task of emptying his bladder, he solved the problem by finding a tube to urinate into. He then collected a number of metal or wooden tubes to help facilitate urination and kept his tubes with him wherever he went.

In a posthypnotic suggestion, Erickson urged the man to find a twelve-inch bamboo tube for urinating. He was to mark it on the outside in quarter-inches. He was told exactly how to hold the tube and how to hold the shaft of his penis. Erickson mentioned that in a day or two, or a week or two, he might consider how long the bamboo needed to be and whether or not he could saw off a quarter-inch, a half-inch, or even one full inch. Erickson explained there was no pressure to do this and he could simply wonder what day of the week he might reduce the length of bamboo. The man was told that he would not be accepted into military service at the present, but arrangements would be made to have him called up in three months' time for a special psychiatric examination. Erickson assured the man he was confident that he would be accepted at that time. The man was then given a total amnesia for the trance experience.

About three months later, the young man was sent to Erickson by the local draft board. He explained that he had been astonished and bewildered to find himself buying bamboo. Then he suddenly remembered Erickson's instructions and felt both embarrassed and hopeful that he could solve his problem. After a week, he sawed off the first inch from the tube. By Thursday he sawed off another two inches. By the end of the month he had only a quarter-inch ring of bamboo left. While using it one day, he realized that the fingers around the shaft of his penis gave him a natural tube. So he discarded the remains of the original bamboo and took great delight in urinating freely and comfortably.

(Erickson, 1954/2001)

A unique aspect of Erickson's work was that he did not believe it was *always* necessary to know why a problem existed or what had caused it. Erickson thought that many behavioral problems were merely habitual patterns of behavior that had outlived their original purpose. This thinking was a radical departure from the analytic therapies of his time, which sought to understand the causal variables behind problem behaviors. Erickson's outcome studies did not support the analytic hypothesis that, if the root cause of a problem is ignored, new symptoms will re-emerge to replace the old ones (Erickson, 1964a). And, unlike the behaviorists, Erickson did not believe that all behavior serves a situationally defined function. Although Erickson would often look for the specific situational antecedents of a behavior, he did not *always* view the immediate environmental consequences as the primary force sustaining the behavior. Instead he sought to understand the subjective meaning of the behavior. As Erickson explained, there is a "need to judge behavior according to the purposes it serves for the specific person" (Erickson, 1941/2001a, p. 4). This understanding includes a recognition of the fact that many problem behaviors are simply learned behaviors based on some chance occurrence in early childhood, which are then maintained by force of habit (Erickson, 1940a/2001).

As early as the 1930s, Erickson devised a technique for dealing with certain types of behavioral problems: those that lacked an immediate situational reinforcer or that produced no appreciable secondary gains. Rather than attempt to directly eliminate a problem behavior, Erickson would gradually introduce some minor change into the behavioral sequence, which would eventually result in a total collapse of the symptom complex. As Erickson explained to his students in a 1936 lecture at Wayne State University College of Medicine, when there are "maladies, whether psychogenic or organic, followed by definite patterns of some sort ... a disruption of this pattern could be a most therapeutic measure; and that it often mattered little how small the disruption was, if introduced early enough" (Erickson, 1936/2001, p.3). This technique would later come to be known as *pattern interruption* (O'Hanlon, 1987).

Although it certainly involves utilization (see Chapter 12), pattern interruption is best understood in light of the strategy of progression. Just like a boat that is gently nudged from its original course, pattern interruption does not require a full and immediate cessation of behavior. Instead the patient is encouraged to keep doing what he or she is already doing but with some slight alteration. Over time, the alterations in the pattern become larger and larger, until finally the pattern is transformed. As Erickson explains, "try to do something that induces a change in the patient ... any little change, because the patient wants a change, however small, and he will accept that as change ... And the change will develop in accord with his own needs" (Gordon and Meyers-Anderson, 1981, pp. 16–17). Erickson called this the "snowball effect." When a snowball is rolled down hill, no one knows exactly where it will go or what it will pick up. It is certain only that the snowball will grow and its path will change.

Patients typically welcome this gradual, progressive approach because, while they may not be certain that they can stop the problem behavior, they are certain of their ability to continue doing it. The case example above illustrates this very well. The patient knew for a fact that he must urinate through a tube. Therefore Erickson instructed him to urinate through a tube, but not the type to which he had become accustomed. Erickson introduced a bamboo tube that was *longer* than his old tubes. These small changes eventually led to the most crucial adjustment, the gradual reduction in the length of the tube. The man was given the opportunity to progressively alter his pattern by marking the tube at quarter-inch intervals. He was never asked to do anything beyond his subjective level of comfort. Progress was inevitable as long as the new therapeutic direction was maintained.

When considering this technique, an important question to ask is why all problem behaviors do not suddenly collapse when met with interruptions. After all, slight deviations of habit can occur naturally on a day-to-day basis. *Pattern interruption is not therapeutic unless it is tied to a systematic process of progression.* Another crucial component of pattern interruption is motivation. If patients are sufficiently motivated to rid themselves of a symptomatic behavior, it is not necessary to study the antecedents and consequences prior to introducing pattern interruption and therapeutic progression. The task of the practitioner is to offer the type of interruption that has some sort of intellectual or emotional appeal. If the patient is curious about the new way of "doing" the problem behavior, or finds the alteration somehow rewarding, then the original pattern is likely to diminish. Like a fissure spreading across a wall, the therapeutic intervention gradually grows, disrupting the established pattern.

An important question to consider is when and where to start the pattern interruption. In most cases, it is best to begin in the office. When possible, Erickson liked to observe a demonstration of the patient's problem behavior. At minimum, he would gain a very detailed verbal account of it. This analysis enabled him to recognize patterns, the responses that were conditioned and highly predictable. After deciding he had a good understanding of a particular behavior, Erickson would then test various small ways it might be manipulated. If the problem was a migraine headache, he would test to see if he could suggest the pain occur in a different anatomical location. If the location could not be altered, he might investigate to see if the onset could be delayed by ten minutes, or five minutes, or even one. If not, he might inquire to see if the headache could be experienced one minute longer than usual, etc. If the patient continues to reject the possibility of maintaining even the slightest alteration, for instance asking a person who smokes 82 cigarettes a day to smoke one cigarette fewer, then it might be necessary to re-examine the patient's commitment to change. Perhaps there are secondary gains or other areas that need to be investigated. Once the patient has experienced some amount of success, under the care and guidance of the practitioner, the changes are generalized to daily living by introducing a progressive interruption into the natural environment.

The elimination of a habitual pattern of behavior is the beginning of the patient's discovery of previously unrecognized potentials. Creating a climate of discovery and experimentation in which any response is accepted as meaningful reduces the danger of the patient's experiencing failure. The type of alteration is not as important as the fact that some sort of interruption is achieved. Greater control is initiated as the patient finds the freedom to respond differently to events and to make choices (Erickson-Klein, 1990). Behavioral alterations commonly used by students of Erickson include postponing or changing the frequency of the behavior's repetitions, changing the objects used in a compulsive ritual, changing the order of the pattern, or changing the location of the behavior (O'Hanlon, 1987, pp. 36–7). In the end, it is the creation of hope and the discovery of new opportunities that matter most.

Cognitive progression

Case report: Maw

Early in his career Erickson was asked to see a 70-year-old woman who went by the name "Maw." She was born in 1860 to parents who did not believe in education for women. At age fourteen she married a sixteen-year-old boy whose formal education was limited to signing checks and "figgering." During the next six years

97

she was kept busy with farm work and pregnancies. As Maw explained, "I learned to figger in my head." But she found it impossible to write any numbers or to sign her name. Maw resented her lack of education and wanted to learn to read.

When she was twenty, Maw had the idea of furnishing room and board for the local schoolteacher. She offered reduced rates in exchange for instruction in reading and writing. Over the next fifty years, many teachers came and left. Each diligently attempted to teach Maw to read and write, but each eventually abandoned the task as hopeless. Maw wanted desperately to read and write. She boarded as many as four teachers at a time, but none succeeded in teaching her. Her children went through grade school, high school, and college. They, too, tried to instruct their mother but without success.

The nature of this impasse seemed to be psychological. As Erickson explained, "It was not that Maw was unintelligent. She had an excellent memory, good critical judgment, listened well, and was remarkably well informed. She often gave strangers … the impression that she had a college education, despite her faulty grammar." However, during her lessons she responded like a small frightened child with a blank mind. As some of her teachers told Erickson, "No matter what you say or do, she just sits there with those eager, troubled eyes, trying hard to make sense out of the nonsense you seem to be saying to her."

While meeting with Erickson, Maw explained, "My son that graduated from engineering school told me that I've got the right gears for reading and writing, but that they are of different sizes, and that's the reason they don't mesh. Now you can file them down or trim them to size because I've got to learn to read and write. Even boarding three teachers and baking and cooking and washing and ironing for them ain't half enough work for me, and I get so tired sitting around with nothing to do. Can you learn me?"

Erickson accepted her as a patient and promised that she would be reading and writing within three weeks, but without being taught anything that she did not already know and had known for a long time. She was puzzled by the statement but eager to cooperate. Erickson continued to emphasize the point that he would not teach her anything she did not already know and had known for a long time. Then she was given paper and pencil and told, "Do not write … just pick up the pencil any old way and hold it in your hand any old way. You and I know you can do that. Any baby can pick up a pencil in any old way." After she had responded Erickson told her, "Now make a mark on the paper, any old scribbling mark like a baby that can't write makes. Just any old crooked mark! That's something you don't even have to learn. Okay. Now make a straight mark on the paper, like you make with a nail when you want to saw a board straight or with a stick when you mark a row in the garden. You can make it short or long or straight up and down or just lying down." After some practice Erickson explained, "Now all those marks you made you can make different sizes and in different places on the paper and in different order and even one on top of the other or one next to another." Erickson then sent her home to practice making more marks stating, "You don't have to believe that it is writing."

The next day she was then shown a neat copy of the "marks" she had made the previous day and was asked to select those that could be used to make a small-scale "rough plan" of the side of a 40-foot barn and to "mark out" such a plan. She was then asked to "split it in the middle" and then to "mark out one 20-foot side of a barn up on top of another one the same size." Bewildered, she did so. Erickson continued to instruct her in this manner carefully maneuvering her into forming all the letters of the alphabet, which were then sequenced together to form small words. Maw was both excited and pleased when Erickson suddenly compared her marks to a child's textbook. Rather than comparing her letters to those in the book, he validated the symbols in the book by showing *their* similarity to *her* constructions, a small but highly significant difference.

In the following days she learned "letter building" and "word building" and "naming." No mention was made of writing or reading. Erickson would say, "Take some of these straight or crooked lines and build me another letter. Now build me a few letters alongside of each other and name the word." Maw was told that, "a dictionary is not a book to read. It is a book to look up words in, just like a picture book isn't for reading, it's just to look at pictures." With the dictionary she was able to discover that she could use vertical, horizontal, oblique, or curved lines to "build" any word in it. Erickson then had her "build" some words taken from the dictionary. She thought the words had been chosen at random and was astonished when Erickson asked her to "name" them. The words were, "Get going Maw and put some grub on the table." Maw declared, "Why, that's what Pa always says—it's just like talking."

After three weeks of lessons, Maw was spending every spare minute with her dictionary and a *Readers' Digest*. She became a prolific reader and a frequent letter writer to her children and grandchildren. Maw lived ten more years before dying of a cerebral hemorrhage.

(Erickson, 1959/2001)

When parents are asked by their toddler, "What does the word 'accident' mean?" they answer, "It means it was not on purpose." But then there is the task of explaining "on purpose," which is difficult if the child does not understand the contrasting concept. Once the child can understand intentions, or purpose, then he can understand accidents. But how do you communicate either idea without having the other as a starting point?

The acquisition of new cognitive constructs requires a preparation of the mind's receptive abilities by starting with familiar background knowledge. New insights are built on top of old understandings that are experiential in nature. A father might say to his child, "Yesterday when you dropped your ice cream on the floor— that was an accident. You did not want it to fall down. When you picked the ice cream up off the ground and put it back on your cone—that was on purpose because you wanted to eat it." In other words, you employ multiple events from past experiences; you use several individual pieces of life learning, and progressively construct a new understanding.

The Socratic Method is an example of cognitive progression that illustrates the timelessness of this technique. Socrates skillfully developed his logical arguments by starting with the other person's answers to his initial questions. This way the final conclusion was based on his audience's understandings rather than Socrates' own background knowledge. Similarly, skillful teachers will often introduce a new idea using concepts that are familiar to the student. This is a form of progression in which recognition of the individual's background knowledge becomes the first crucial step.

Within the context of therapy, it is often helpful to introduce alternative explanations for events or to create entirely new realities. However, the words of the practitioner have little meaning if the appropriate cognitive structures are not already in place. Similar to a young learner, patients sometimes need to be *primed* for new thinking using familiar elements from their experiential past. When you simply introduce key words, a person's receptivity to ideas that reflect these words is significantly increased. In the same way that a gas engine is primed with fuel, so that it will start more easily, research has shown that new associational networks develop with greater ease when verbal priming has taken place (Wann and Branscombe, 1990).

This is illustrated in the case above as Erickson used language and images from the farm to prime Maw for the task of decoding words. Maw was capable of doing calculation in her head so Erickson described the dimension of a barn gable to form the letter "A." She was able to look at and identify pictures in books so Erickson described the combination of symbols in a dictionary as images with names. All of the new activities were provided within the context of her past experiential learnings and introduced in a slow progressive manner.

Another frequent challenge to therapeutic progress occurs when the patient lacks the emotional readiness to hear disturbing ideas. This common phenomenon is reflected in the statement, "Your words have fallen on deaf ears." Psychological constructs, such as denial, have been used to describe the mind's ability to stubbornly block any reality it is not ready to process. But there are ways to get around this sort of barrier.

Erickson devised a method for progressively introducing information, which he termed *seeding*. In the way that seeds are planted in the ground for future harvest, Erickson would begin to lay the foundation for an important therapeutic idea by casually inserting related concepts earlier in the session or even during prior sessions. The technique is similar to "foreshadowing," which is a literary tool used to prepare the mind for some dramatic point in the story. For a patient, the impending insight might be a frightening reality such as recognizing that a loved one is terminally ill, or it could be a life-altering event such as learning that one is about to become a parent. It is often slow progression that makes assimilation of emotionally loaded ideas more likely. During this time, other associations are made so that the new reality has support and can be acted on in a way that is helpful.

Rather than attempting to force a memory or idea on the patient, careful seeding allows the patient to develop the thinking on his or her own. When used appropriately, it is a respectful and gentle technique. The following example comes from one of Short's earliest experiences with hypnosis. The woman he was preparing to hypnotize asked if she could lie on the floor while he performed the induction. Short agreed and noticed that she lay on her back with her legs stiff and her arms folded across her chest, as though she were in a casket. He asked her what she wanted to visualize during the trance and she said, "A vacation on the river with my husband. It is something we do every year." Short complied with her request and focused on memories of enjoyable times on the river, people who were greatly valued, and the experience of moments we all want to last forever. The trance lasted for approximately twenty minutes. Short concluded the exercise with the following statement, "This has been a relaxing and wonderful experience but all good things must come to an end."

Hearing this, the woman burst into tears and wept profusely. Observers in the room were bewildered because she had been smiling throughout the trance experience. After a few moments, she regained her composure and politely thanked Short for helping her come to terms with her husband's impending death. She said that, although the doctors had told her that his heart would not last much longer, she had not been able to accept the imminent reality of this terrible loss. The trance had given her the opportunity of once again traveling down the river with him, even though he was not physically present. She explained that, now that she was no longer in a state of denial, she could begin making necessary arrangements. The experiential exercise had provided a safe gradual progression toward a moment of "awakening."

Forward progression

Case report: The woman who was considering an affair

A woman who had recently learned of her husband's affair came to Erickson for advice. She had just discovered her husband had had sex with another woman in their apartment complex. She was both hurt and filled with rage. She was contemplating revenge and told Erickson that she had noticed a handsome man down the hall who was giving her the eye. She wanted Erickson to tell her whether she should have an affair in order to "get back" at her husband.

Erickson explained that the answer was already in her unconscious mind and that he would use hypnosis so that he might know what the answer is. After teaching her time distortion, Erickson had her go forward in time to a point after having the purposed affair. The woman described herself as being horribly depressed and lost in despair. She explained that after having the affair she experienced a tremendous loss of self-respect and was more troubled by her misbehavior than her husband had been by his. Furthermore, she realized that he no longer had to feel guilty for his actions since she was just as culpable. In the trance, the woman pleaded with Erickson to convince her conscious mind that she must not have this affair. So Erickson woke her from trance and related everything she had said to him in trance. The woman thanked Erickson. She said that she had her answer and that she would use her husband's guilt to reconcile her own feelings of anger

(Erickson, 1977a)

When a person becomes paralyzed by indecision or overwhelming emotions, therapeutic progress requires an activation of the will. But first of all the person must know what it is that he or she wants. If the practitioner can persuade the patient to think about a desired outcome, then significant progress is made toward having him or her actualize it. That is why so many schools of therapy now include the practice of therapeutic contracting. This is a technique by which therapeutic goals are clarified. When viewed from the perspective of progression, it is easy to see how defining concrete aspects of a positive outcome facilitates improvement.

Forward progression is a technique in which patients mentally go forward in time in order to recognize some desired outcome (see also "Reorientation in time," on p. 175). This might be accomplished by asking patients to think forward to a period of time after the problem has been resolved and to speculate about the details. The exercise takes on a greater experiential quality when hypnotic elements are added. For instance, the therapist might ask the patient who wants to have a family in ten years, "How does it feel to be in this family? What do the children look like? What does the house look like? What smells are in the house? What noises do you hear in the home?" By having this sort of ideosensory experience, patients are given a pleasing vision that provides a sense of direction and increased motivation, and are thus less likely to remain immobilized.

A technique used frequently in solution-focused therapy and cognitive behavioral therapy is *self-anchored scaling*. This quantitative technique is used to assign a number to subjective realities. For instance, a person who is experiencing fear might be asked to rate the fear on a scale of one to ten. Next the patient is asked what he or she could do to bring the number up (or down) by just one point, or even by half a point. This creates a slow progression forward as the patient endeavors to imagine the possibility of experiencing slight improvement.

When working with extremely neurotic patients, who cannot imagine even the smallest amount of progress, a therapist can begin the scaling exercise using negative integers as the starting point. The next question is, "What would it take to get you from a negative five to a negative four?" The question enables the person to consider a future in which some small amount of progress has been achieved but without having to commit to "actual" change. If the person cannot make any statements about how they want the future to be, then they can be asked to pretend the knowledge is there. This again reduces the amount of commitment while still achieving some progress. After this beginning step has been accomplished, and the patient begins to feel more comfortable, then he or she is ready for the next small step, which is usually some form of concrete action.

In the case of the woman whose husband had an affair, hypnosis was used to allow access to a different emotional state. In the future, after her revenge had been achieved, she would no longer have the feelings of rage that were currently clouding her judgment. Most importantly, the decision of what to do came from her self-understandings rather than from the clinician's judgment. This set the proper conditions for *her* to maintain responsibility for *her* behavior. And as Erickson was fond of saying, independence is a primary joy of life.

The general application of progression

The logic of progression applies to any effort to introduce new behavior or thinking. Like the elasticity of the body, the psychological structure of the mind can be reshaped and new behaviors produced but there are limits on how much stretching can be done at a single moment in time. Both the mind and body need time to adjust.

Questions of clinical judgment that are dictated by this type of logic might be, "How much change is the patient going to be able to accept at this time?" or "At what pace can therapy progress without overwhelming this person?" The answers to these important questions are sometimes obvious, though the situation may be complex. A woman who is in an unhealthy relationship might say to the therapist, "I just can't imagine the possibility of leaving him." Using good clinical judgment, the therapist would delay an apparently necessary discussion about her getting out of the relationship. An appropriate place to start would be things that she *can* imagine. A good first step might be to have her describe, in detail, the various things that she needs and wants from *life*, rather than focusing directly on the problematic relationship. The next step might be to describe the things her children need from her, while they are still young and *living* at home.[1] This progression of ideas might occur over the course of one hour or over a period of months. Ideally, it is the patient who determines the pace at which

[1] Of course, if the partner is threatening the welfare of the children, then there is a duty to warn. Unfortunately, this reality would have to be forced on the patient during the session when it becomes apparent and a report made to Child Protective Services.

change will occur, though sometimes it is the situation that determines what the clinician must attempt to communicate. Whenever
a practitioner begins to sense a great deal of resistance, then it is
time to reassess the patient's immediate needs.

The implications of this strategy are both obvious and subtle.
When one is sitting down to talk with a person it makes sense to
start with less threatening topics and gradually progress to more
distressing topics. This is an important skill with application in
many different settings. For example, the pediatrician Sanghavi
(2003) describes a semistructured method for eliciting information
from adolescents. The acronym HEADSS helps the practitioner
remember the order in which topics are approached. First there is
a discussion of life at *home*, then the adolescent's *educational* experiences or employment, then a discussion of his favorite *activities*,
then there are questions about *drug* use, *sexual* behavior, and
finally the topic of *suicide* or depression is discussed. This simple
approach provides a semistructured interview that is both comprehensive and likely to elicit information. Describing a case in
which he used the technique, Sanghavi writes, "Progressively, we
explored Jasper's high-risk behaviors ... Surprisingly, it was easy
to get him to talk" (pp. 197–8). The conversation was "easy"
because it was conducted in a skillful way.

It is an automatic function of the mind to keep the flow of conscious awareness away from ideas that are likely to overwhelm the
system. Therefore, when one is speaking to patients the conversation should start with something that is clearly tolerable. If
patients need to discuss a painful childhood experience, then they
should be invited to begin with a benign memory. Or, as Erickson
would say, "If they cannot tolerate a full remembrance, then you
can ask them what part of it they can stand to remember today;
and what part they can stand to remember tomorrow" (Erickson,
1955a).

While one is coming to a better understanding of the strategy of
progression, the less obvious implication is the importance of
good assessment. In order for this strategy to succeed, it is necessary to identify and target a highly stable aspect of the symptom
complex. If the practitioner attempts to make small steps forward
in an area of behavior that the patient already feels free to alter,

then there is less likelihood that therapy will be seen as useful. However, if the problem always occurs in a certain way and this is what is altered, then the therapy is validated. For instance, while working with a migraine headache, Erickson might learn that it occurs every ten days, in the morning, without fail. In that instance, he might attempt to delay the onset by one or two hours. If the headache always occurred behind the left eye, then he might attempt to alter its location. If the headaches always lasted for five full hours, he might attempt to reduce it to four hours and fifty-five minutes. In other words, the assessment needs to contain questions about symptom intensity, frequency, duration, and time of onset. As the patient begins to reconfigure his or her thinking about the negative expectancies, new opportunities are created for the discovery of previously unrecognized abilities.

Another subtle application of progression can be made when a given treatment does not appear to be working. The effectiveness of any healing ritual can sometimes be enhanced by increasing its "dose" or by repeating the intervention in such a way that suggests greater therapeutic potency to the patient (Kirsch, 1990, p. 51).

As with all of the clinical strategies described in this volume, progression can be misapplied. The strategy is not likely to work if the therapist is working toward a goal that is of little value to the patient. Because it is sometimes a slow process, motivation is crucial for progression to succeed. The *patient* must really want to arrive at the final destination toward which the small steps are being directed.

Furthermore, there must be careful consideration of what is the next most appropriate step for this individual. Again, using the example of a woman in an abusive relationship, if she has become hypervigilant, unable to sleep for days, and is now feeling that she is going crazy, due to sleep deprivation, then the first step is help her restore her ability to sleep. If she has become ill over a period of days and has been unable to hold down food or water, then the first step would be to help her obtain medical attention. These examples illustrate the fact that sometimes the first step may not seem directly related to the psychotherapeutic objective. However, as Erickson would often say, the clinician needs to be mindful of the patient as a total creature (Erickson, 1955a). While asking the question, "What is the next thing that this person needs to be able to do?" there should be a developing awareness of the patient's immediate needs, whether psychological, physical, or social. While keeping an eye to the final objective, the practitioner must not forget to take into account the vehicle of progress.

Chapter 10

Suggestion

This chapter provides a glimpse into the strategy for which Erickson was considered the undisputed master. It is almost impossible to talk about Erickson's contribution to the fields of medicine and psychotherapy without making reference to his use of suggestion. Unfortunately, suggestion is often subsumed within a discussion of hypnosis as if to imply that its value is inextricably linked to the hypnotic protocol. While this chapter addresses the use of hypnosis more than any other, the focus continues to remain on the broader principles underlying Erickson's methodology. As will be seen in the following case examples, suggestion is by no means limited to the application of a single procedure.

Case report: The boy with asthma

Erickson was brought a twelve-year-old boy who suffered from chronic asthma. The boy had to have an inhaler with him at all times. As Erickson began speaking with the boy he noticed the number of times the boy reached for his inhaler so that he could breathe comfortably. The boy was obviously anxious. So Erickson asked sympathetically, "How much fear do you have of asthma … how intense is this fear?" Erickson listened quietly, without making any attempt to assure the boy. Instead, he had him elaborate on his subjective experiences of asthma: "How important are your fears of arrested breathing?" The boy responded with noticeable relief. This was the first time anybody had ever wanted to listen to a full account of his fears about death and of arrested breathing. The boy became absorbed in conversation with Erickson. He explained in full detail his fear of suddenly becoming unable to breath. He described the horrible feeling of constriction in his chest and the awful visions of death that came to him. In telling his story, he became so fascinated by at last having a good listener that he began breathing more comfortably.

When Erickson felt that the boy was ready to accept the suggestion, he pointed out, "You know … talking about your fear makes it easier for you to breathe." The boy acknowledged that this was true. So Erickson continued, "I would like to have you understand that some of your asthma is caused by fear and some of it comes from the pollen. You take the medication that you do in order to deal with the part of the asthma that is caused by the pollen. Now let us say that you currently have one hundred percent asthma, if I reduce that asthma by one percent, you won't notice the change. But your asthma would be one percent less." Next, Erickson speculated, "Suppose I reduce the asthma by two percent … five percent … or ten percent. You still wouldn't notice the change but it would have been reduced." Erickson spoke in such a way as to get the boy curious about the idea of reducing the asthma by some unspecified amount.

He then engaged the boy in a debate over just how much of the asthma he was going to keep. "Is it going to be five percent … or ten percent … or twenty percent … or thirty percent … or forty percent?" The boy decided, "I think it is twenty percent of the asthma that comes from the pollen." This gave him the freedom to use his inhaler eighty percent less than before.

(Erickson, 1965b)

"Know that I and thou and the disease are three factors mutually antagonistic. If thou wilt side with me, not neglecting what I enjoin on thee and refraining from such things as I shall forbid thee, then we shall be two against one and will overcome the disease."
– unnamed physician, c. 1200 CE

The use of suggestion in healing has existed since antiquity. Ancient Greeks and Egyptians and Oriental cultures are known to have used rituals to elicit behavioral responses outside the normal realm of conscious control. These included, among other things, the curing of disease and removal of demons, which by today's standards would be recognized as the restoration of sanity. As would be expected, the dramatic results achieved through suggestion have time and again inspired both profound respect and intense mistrust. In the current culture, it is not uncommon for critics to dismiss clinical techniques of suggestion as being insincere or overly manipulative. Before becoming comfortable with the use of suggestion in therapy, the clinician must first come to terms with the loneliness and desperation associated with intractable suffering. From this perspective it is easier to appreciate *the essential function of clinical suggestion,* which *is to help the patient accomplish a goal that consciously he cannot reach alone.*

In 1994, members of the North Texas Society for Clinical Hypnosis had the opportunity to listen to an accomplished general surgeon, Dabney Ewin, lecture on his work with industrial burn victims. In an interview conducted two years later, Ewin explained:

> When I started using hypnosis with burn victims, I was convinced at first that the burns simply were not as severe as I had originally diagnosed, but shortly thereafter, I treated a patient whose leg had slipped into molten metal at an aluminum plant. Using hypnosis I had him [become] "cool and comfortable" a half hour after his burn, and when he got out of the hospital in 18 days, without a skin graft and without narcotics, I became a true believer.

> (Ewin, 1996, p. 18)

At the lecture in Dallas, after watching an intriguing series of slides documenting the uses of suggestion for providing relief from pain, reducing inflammation, speeding up recovery, and reducing the severity of scarring, a member of the audience suddenly asked, "What is your method of hypnotic induction?" Ewin replied, "I typically meet my patients at the door of the ER. They come in strapped to a gurney and packed in ice. I tell them I am a doctor and emphatically ask if *they* know how to stop their pain. When they say 'No,' I tell them that I *do.* Then I ask if they are willing to do *everything* I ask. When they say 'Yes,' I tell them to feel cool all over their body, and to keep on feeling cool as they are wheeled into their room."

Ewin pointed out that this is not such an extraordinary suggestion because the patient is already packed in ice. Yet typically, with the supplemental use of suggestion, much less pain medication is required and healing is greatly facilitated (Ewin, 1996). This acceptance of what the patient knows he cannot do and the offering of hope through direct suggestion gives the patient a needed ally in dealing with his fear and pain.

During the last century, the therapeutic use of suggestion has been closely associated with the practice of hypnosis. In 1842, James Braid introduced the terms "hypnotism" and "hypnosis" from the Greek *hypnos* (sleep) to describe a special state of consciousness that he believed was associated with heightened responsiveness to suggestion. Forty years later, Hippolyte Bernheim would identify suggestion as the sole operative force in hypnotism (Hughes and Rothovius, 1996). In modern times, most people agree that hypnotic results are achieved by means of suggestion. A general definition, purposed by Weitzenhoffer (1989), describes hypnotism as "a form of influence by one person exerted on another through the medium or agency of suggestion" (p. 13). Accordingly, much of the literature on hypnosis seeks to delineate the exact means by which increased suggestibility is best achieved. But, beyond this, opinions become widely divergent and there continues to be controversy over what exactly is hypnosis (Short, 1999).

As one of the originators of the modern practice of hypnosis, Braid emphasized the importance of hypnotic induction by using a shiny object to produce eye fatigue. At this time, sleep was believed to play a central role in suggestibility. Braid proposed that, "The patient must be made to understand that he is to keep the eyes steadily fixed on the object, and *the mind riveted on the idea* [our emphasis] of that one object" (Hughes and Rothovius, 1996, p. 136). Bernheim later recognized that therapeutic suggestion *does not necessarily require induction into hypnotic sleep to be effective*. This discovery in the nineteenth century by Bernheim anticipated the general use of suggestion in psychotherapy, a form of therapy that had yet to be invented by twentieth-century psychotherapists.

As a college student, Erickson essentially accepted the Braidian explanation of hypnosis but would soon downplay the importance of external objects and formal induction rituals. He instead placed great emphasis on the fixation of attention on a single idea. Erickson clarified his unique clinical approach to suggestion stating that,

Innumerable times this author has been asked to commit to print in detail the hypnotic technique he has employed to alleviate intolerable pain or to correct various other problems. The verbal replies made to these many requests have never seemed to be adequate since they were invariably prefaced by the earnest assertion that the technique in itself serves no other purpose than that of securing and *fixating the attention of patients, creating then a receptive and responsive mental state*, and thereby enabling them to *benefit from unrealized or only partially realized potentials* [our emphasis] for behavior of various types. With this achieved by the hypnotic technique, there is then the opportunity to proffer suggestions and instructions serving to aid and to direct patients in achieving the desired goal or goals. In other words, the hypnotic technique serves only to induce a favorable setting in which to instruct patients in a more advantageous use of their own potentials of behavior.

(Erickson, 1966/2001, p.1)

Before attempting an in-depth study of Erickson's use of suggestion, it is important to recognize that, while the concept of suggestion is indispensable to the theory of hypnosis, the use of suggestion is not limited to the formal procedures of hypnosis.

The person who originated the concept of clinical suggestion, Bernheim, defined therapeutic suggestion in very broad terms, as, "the aptitude to transform an *idea* [our emphasis] into an act" (recall Erickson's discovery of ideomotor movement when as a teenager he spontaneously transformed the idea of motion into the act of rocking the chair to which he was strapped). The first English translation of Bernheim's use of suggestion in healing was printed in 1897 and entitled *Suggestive Therapeutics* (Hughes and Rothovius, 1996, p. 173). However, over half a century would pass before the field as a whole came to realize that hypnosis is not the only form of therapy in which suggestion functions as the central strategy.

Beginning in the 1950s, placebo therapies began to be studied as another form of suggestive therapeutics. A placebo can be any medical treatment that contains no active ingredients or certifiable remedial action. There are placebo pills as well as placebo surgery. One early study found that placebo surgery for bleeding ventricular and duodenal ulcers was far more effective than active surgery

(Volgyesi, 1954). Similarly, Thomsen, et al. (1983) found that placebo surgery for Ménière's disease produced a 77% success rate, with active surgery having only a 70% success rate. Whether pill or surgery, the placebo merely creates an aptitude toward the *idea* that healing is likely to occur. Placebo treatment is now broadly recognized as being capable of producing genuine curative effects (Kirsch, 1990).

In a landmark text, written by Jerome Frank (1973) on the topic of social influence, the observation was made that most psychotherapy patients suffer from a sense of helplessness, hopelessness, and demoralization. According to Frank, effective therapies enhance patients' positive expectations, restore their faith in the future, and foster a sense of mastery and competence. The restoration of hope, says Frank, is the curative factor in psychotherapy. This perspective helped open the way for the incorporation of suggestion into hope- and competency-based models of therapy (Snyder, 2000; Waters and Lawrence, 1993). After all, what is hope if it does not, at a minimum; contain the implicit suggestion that things can get better.

Because almost any form of communication can result in suggestion, its precise boundaries are difficult to establish. One might even go so far as to argue that clinical suggestion occurs any time the therapist elicits a response from the patient that somehow exceeds the bounds of what the patient believed to be possible prior to therapy. What is clear is that all of the clinician's words and actions can potentially suggest something to the patient and such suggestions can have a powerful effect. That is why it is important to recognize this strategy as something to be applied with careful intention. As stated by Erickson,

> It's awfully important, if you want to deal with patients with organic illness or psychogenic illness, that you *know what you say* and *what the implications of what you say are* [our emphasis]. How they extend into the future and how they reach into the past and how they modify the present and how they convey understandings by the natural elaboration in terms of their own thinking that occurs when you speak.

> (Erickson, 1965c)

In regard to the boy with asthma, it is clear that Erickson used partitioning in support of the clinical suggestion. He communicated the *idea* that some relief from asthma was possible. This idea was eventually transformed into action. Did this use of suggestion constitute hypnosis? There is no mention by Erickson of a hypnotic induction, yet he was very careful to build up the situation and wait until the right moment to offer the idea that the boy had an unrealized ability to control his asthma. Erickson began by creating an intense inward focus of attention. He fully absorbed the boy in his thoughts by making an earnest inquiry into the boy's emotional experience with asthma. He listened to all of the boy's fears and communicated a sympathetic understanding of the boy's situation. The clinical suggestion he offered was very direct: you have begun to breathe more comfortably therefore you can control some portions of your asthma. Similar to Ewin's failure-proof suggestion that a person packed in ice can feel cool, Erickson was offering an idea that matched the boy's immediate experience. The boy recognized that he did not feel as frightened while speaking with Erickson and as a result he was breathing more easily. This is the type of response that would be expected because now the boy had an ally. As soon as Erickson began to listen sympathetically, and as he began to speculate on what *"we"* can do about the asthma, the boy was no longer forced to face his disease alone.

Finally, it should be recognized that, although Erickson's suggestion was targeted at symptom reduction, this was not the only achievement. By overcoming this frightening problem the boy learned a lot about his own resiliencies. Erickson's general approach to problem solving was to use the amelioration of symptoms as the being of a snowball effect leading to the reorganization of ideas about self, others, and the environment (Zeig and Geary, 1990). As Erickson commented on this case, "It completely altered the boy's attitude toward life" (Erickson, 1965b).

Cooperation versus control

Case report: The woman who was going to slap Erickson

A young woman walked into Erickson's office and glared at him. Her husband had arranged the appointment. Erickson greeted her by saying, "Your husband has told me that if I say a *single* wrong word here that you will slap my face and walk out." Erickson continued with an earnest tone, "There is just one thing puzzling me ... I don't know which way to duck. Are you right or left handed?" Startled, she looked at Erickson. "Maybe you won't say the wrong thing," she said. Erickson acknowledged her statement: "Maybe I won't." But then he added, "Well, you are my height. You are very nicely built. You weigh quite a bit less than I do and I'm not very heavy. You are as tall as I am. But none the less, you could really swing. So are you right or left handed?" She replied, "Right handed." From that point forward, Erickson was able to gather further information about her therapeutic needs, without being slapped.

(Erickson, 1962d)

Above all else, it should be recognized that Erickson's strategic use of suggestion was not for purposes of control but rather as a means of collecting and guiding the patient's expenditure of energy. Using hypnosis to facilitate an intense inward focus of attention, Erickson would then guide the patient to a confident and sustained recognition of his own potential for healing. An analogy for this approach to healing can be seen in the riddle, "How do you start a daytime fire using only what is found in the air?" It is not often that daylight catches things on fire so why expect it to happen? But, when a magnifying glass is introduced and gathers ordinary light into a small focused point on paper, without movement, a flame develops. In just the same way, people often achieve extraordinary outcomes using ordinary everyday actions, once their energy is focused and held consistently to the task at hand.

The strategic use of suggestion can produce some stunning results. When seemingly improbable outcomes are associated with the actions of an authority figure, it is not surprising that the illusion of control exists. As described by Erickson, "By acceptance of and response to suggestions, the subject can become psychologically deaf, blind, hallucinate, amnesic, anesthetic or dissociated, or he can develop various special types of behavior regarded by him as reasonable, or desirable in the given situation" (Erickson, 1961/2001a, p. 5). It is important to recognize that, because the behavior *must be regarded by the subject as reasonable*, the operator does not actually have control.

Furthermore, Erickson insisted that all hypnotic behaviors are naturally occurring phenomena. For example, many sports enthusiasts become *psychologically deaf* any time a football game is on TV. After one has watched a very scary movie it is not difficult to *hallucinate* a sight or sound associated with some of the fright produced by the film. Almost everyone has had the experience of being introduced to a person and then five seconds later becoming *amnesic* to the person's name. And anyone who has ever been involved in a thrilling, physically vigorous activity knows that you can become scratched and bruised without recognizing when or how you received the injury. As mentioned above, any of these everyday actions can be summoned and focused with great intensity on a given clinical problem. The results are not a product of control but are instead the result of a cooperative endeavor, an alliance of the patient and clinician against the clinical problem.

While cautioning against the use of hypnosis to satisfy fantasies of control, Erickson warns, "Failures in hypnotic experimentation and therapy often derive from treating the subject as an automaton, expected to execute commands in accord with the hypnotist's understanding, rather than as a personality with individual patterns of response and behavior" (Erickson, 1961/2001a, p. 3). Although hypnotists sometimes use "challenge" suggestions to heighten the patient's expectation of achieving profound clinical results, the outcome is still a product of cooperation. For example, a woman might be told, "You can now realize that your legs have become *immobile*. Just *try* to stand and see what happens." If the situational conditions are right, the patient will find that she is unable to stand. But this is by her choice and must therefore be in accord with her own agenda. The patient might just as easily stand up in order to rebuff the challenge. As Erickson explains, "… no one can predict with utter certainty just how a subject is going to use such stimuli. One names or indicates possible ways, but the subjects behave in accord with their learnings" (Erickson, 1964/2001b, p. 28). This is why, when using suggestion in therapy, it is so important to establish with the patient an adequate understanding of the purpose of the suggestion and how it relates to his or her unique needs (Erickson, Hershman, and Sector, 1961, p. 272).

This section was introduced with a case illustrating a masterful utilization of behavior. As Erickson points out, a woman who tells her husband that she will slap the therapist as soon as he says one single wrong word is not likely to cooperate with therapy. It was the husband who arranged the therapy, leaving her all the more ready to feel self-righteously indignant at anything Erickson had to say, with the exception of hearing herself quoted. When he stated her position, she was forced to agree with him. Having her words quoted most likely also induced some self-consciousness. When he asked her which way he should duck, Erickson made it clear that he was willing to accept her on her terms and cooperate with her actions. In return, he asked her to cooperate with him. As Erickson explains, "Why shouldn't I get cooperation from a girl who promised that to her husband? It is a very important thing to get cooperation" (Erickson, 1962d). She cooperated by revealing to him that she was right-handed. Before that, she cooperated by listening to Erickson as he complimented her body, stating that she was nicely built and that she was not overly heavy, and that she could really swing, which implied strength in her body. As he made these remarks, her focus of attention undoubtedly turned inward, creating a state of mind more responsive to suggestion. She was not under Erickson's control, but was certainly more willing to cooperate.

Direct suggestion

Case report: The mother's unconscious use of direct suggestion

I (Short) was talking about hypnosis with a social worker when she recalled, "I almost got to witness hypnosis first-hand but I had to cancel the appointment at the very last minute. It was really embarrassing." Intrigued, I asked her to explain. She had been trying to get a large wart removed from her son's hand but the pediatrician was unsuccessful in his efforts to remove it. Each time it was treated, the wart reappeared, larger in size. As a last resort, the mother was told to try taking her son to a hypnotist. As she explained, "My son was just eight. I did not want him to be frightened by what was about to happen so each night, before bed, I told him that a nice person was going to talk with him on Saturday to make his wart disappear. We were counting down the days until Saturday, when he was supposed to have his appointment. But when I got him out of bed Saturday morning, the wart was gone!" Many years later she was still baffled. My response was, "You did not get to watch someone else conduct hypnosis on your son. You did it yourself!" She still looked puzzled so I explained, "You failed to mention that he should wait until after he saw the man on Saturday to lose his wart."

Erickson defined suggestion generally as the communication of ideas. Although he did not provide a precise definition of direct suggestion, he seemed to use the term to refer to the classical use hypnotic suggestion. While using traditional approaches to suggestion, ideas are communicated in a linguistic style that is easily evaluated by conscious processes. Direct suggestions usually take on the form of an injunction that clearly originates from some external source, "Your eyes are becoming tired and sleepy, and you will continue to feel more and more tired and sleepy, and soon you will fall into a deep hypnotic sleep!" Under these circumstances there is no doubt over who is giving the commands and who is expected to respond to the ideas. This particular use of suggestion becomes therapeutic when the ideas that are communicated relate to the needs and goals of the patient.

People in general are vulnerable to the verbal influence of others and sometimes to a greater extent than is realized. As a patient once commented to Short, "It is amazing what you find yourself able to do after someone *really* tells you to do it. When I went to army boot camp, I was not physically capable of doing more than ten pushups. After smarting off at the drill sergeant, I suddenly found myself outside, in the rain, doing a hundred pushups over a mud puddle. With him screaming at me I was suddenly able to do far more than before." This was a patient who had an extremely harsh and authoritative father. From a young age he had been programmed to respond to an external locus of control. This was his preference in therapy as well. He was annoyed by other therapists who merely sat and listened. He wanted a therapist who would tell him what to do about his current situation.

Although Erickson is most commonly studied for his use of indi-rect suggestion, he did not hesitate in using direct suggestion when he felt it would be beneficial. Betty Alice Erickson remem-bers as an adolescent being wakened by her father at about 5 a.m. She had just gotten her driver's license and Erickson wanted her to practice by taking a road trip. As she lay in bed complaining about having to get up, Erickson fixed her eyes with his. "Get up. In eighty years you can rest all you want, but right now you are going to get up and enjoy life!" Because she did get out of bed and enjoyed her road trip with her father, Betty Alice committed to the rest of the suggestion, which was to do things to enjoy life for at least the next eighty years. His words remain in her memory as a blessing to this day. This was Erickson's way of using a straight-forward phrase to enter people's consciousness and thereby change their life.

Unfortunately, people do not always offer blessings to others but sometimes use direct suggestion as a curse. As an example, how many times has a new teacher sat in the teacher lounge listening to a more experienced colleague state, "Believe me, you are not going to get anywhere with this child—he will frustrate you until the point that your head begins to throb." For the person who under-stands the power of suggestion, it comes as no surprise when later in the semester the new teacher develops a problem with headaches, which she blames on the student. This responsiveness to suggestion is why it is so unfortunate when a woman who is about to experience her first pregnancy finds herself under the care of a dogged nurse who insists, "You can't be in *real* labor yet. When it starts, you're really going to feel pain. It's going to be the worst pain you have ever felt in your entire life. You're going to beg for the epidural!"

Fortunately, there are many individuals who have a very adequate understanding of suggestion and how it can be used to benefit oth-ers. For instance, the mother who instinctively tells her injured child, "I am going to kiss your boo-boo three times. Each time it will feel a little better. On the third kiss," the mother says with a happy smile, "the pain will go away." Similarly, a mom told her frightened child, "Before you go to your first day of school, I am going to slip a Mommy-Love Ring on your finger. You will have it on your finger all day and it will make you feel safe and happy.

But no one else will be able to see it, because a Mommy-Love Ring is invisible." At that point, an imaginary ring was slipped onto the child's finger, in order to "see if it fits."

When seeking to use suggestion with children, there is reason to believe that direct suggestion will work more effectively than indirect suggestion. While conducting research to compare children's responsiveness to specific and nonspecific instructions, to increase salivary immune substances, it has been found that only those subjects given specific suggestions were able to increase immune substances (Olness, Culbert, and Uden, 1989). This need for specificity has been observed by other experts in child hypnosis. Gardner (1974) has argued that subtle cues intended to direct the child's behavior may be misunderstood by the child, resulting in frustration or an unexpected response. Children obviously do not have the same degree of cognitive sophistication as adults and are also lacking many of the life experiences that bring meaning to the associations adults make. For instance, Gardner (1974) warns that when using suggestion to encourage a child to eat more food, it is sometimes necessary to instruct the child to see, smell, and *eat* specific foods rather than to use a more general suggestion to experience feelings of hunger. The point to be recognized is that the subject, for whom the suggestion is intended, whether young or old, should have a clear understanding of the idea that is being communicated.

A good illustration of the ease in which direct suggestion can be applied is described in a research study (Spanos and Gorassini, 1984) on resiliency to pain. The researchers used two different methods to create pain: one was to submerse the subject's arm in a freezing tank of ice water; the other was to slowly increase the pressure of a blade against the subject's finger. The subjects were asked to endure the painful stimuli for as long as they felt they could stand it. It was discovered during separate trials, with different groups, that subjects could endure greater amounts of painful stimuli without complaint after being told, "Do whatever you can to reduce pain." *Merely receiving explicit permission from the investigator significantly increased the coping resources of the subjects.* A formal hypnotic induction was not necessary for the effect to occur. This finding was interpreted as an indication that hypnotic coping suggestions may produce their effects simply by sanctioning the use of pre-existing capacities. This outcome could also be seen as evidence of increased resiliency, created through the introduction of hope.

Erickson believed that direct injunctions are needed for patients who are in an uncertain state. This would be true of those experiencing physical pain, if they are not certain how much more pain they can take. It would also be true of those who question their readiness for change. Erickson compared this style of suggestion to the type of communication used with children: "... when a child is uncertain about something, you say, 'I'll tell you when to go ... Now!' " (Erickson, Rossi, and Rossi, 1976, p. 169).

The use of a single word, "now," provides much impetus without requiring time and effort for processing. As a general rule, statements that require less effortful processing are more successful in influencing the general evaluations people hold of themselves, other people, objects, and issues (Obermiller, 1985). According to Bernheim, the simpler the suggestions, the more readily they take effect (Hughes and Rothovius, 1996).

As mentioned above, there are certain situations in which direct suggestion is especially useful. These seem to be cases in which the patient suffers from excessive inhibition or self-doubt. When direct suggestion is offered at the right moment, by the right person, there is an external validation of existing motives and capabilities. After all, the stage hypnotist would not be able to get the shy audience member to come up on stage and cluck like a chicken unless the person was wishing for an opportunity to overcome the shyness.

Indirect suggestion

Case report: The tale of two trees

Unfortunately, Erickson was not able to outlive all of the patients who came to him for care. In the final years of his life, Erickson was very involved in preparing his patients, family, and friends for his eventual departure. He knew that it was especially important to make provisions for those who were chronically mental ill, those who had become dependent on therapy in order to live independently. Occasionally some patients benefit from a lifelong relationship with a single therapist.

One such person, John, had begun therapy with Erickson in the early 1960s. He was schizophrenic and had a trust fund established by his family that allowed him to live independently. When driving became difficult for John, Erickson helped him find an apartment within walking distance of his home office. From the very start, John became especially attached to Erickson. John was a kind and faithful person whom Erickson enjoyed having at his home.

A great deal of therapy was achieved with John. One of Erickson's methods was to simultaneously position himself as a powerful authority figure and as one who was one down in relation to the patient's ability. When Erickson decided that John should learn how to be responsible and care for others, he sent him to the pound to get a dog. John's apartment was too small for a dog so Erickson offered to give John's dog, Barney, a home. John came to the Erickson house twice a day to feed and care for Barney. The dog allegedly wrote a series of limericks about his relationship with John and about the "old codger" and how he was "terrorized" by the sight of his wheelchair and honking horn. It was clearly John who became the dog's hero.

(Zeig, 1985)

Erickson and this patient especially enjoyed spending time together outside. A few years before he died, he and John planted two trees in the backyard. It was the beginning of a friendly competition to see whose tree grew stronger and taller.

Several months after Erickson's death, the patient's tree began to wither and die. By this time, the patient had become a dear family friend, a relationship that continues to this day. Mrs. Erickson knew about the "tree competition" and was concerned about the effect that the dying of John's tree might have on him. So she offered to get the weaker tree some help: "Let's have a specialist examine your tree." John was initially befuddled, but then explained, "That is Dr Erickson's tree! Right after we planted them, Dr Erickson decided that he wanted my tree. So we traded."

With pride he pointed to the other tree. "My tree is doing fine. It always has."[1]

Those who knew Erickson recognize him as the undisputed master of indirect communication. Erickson's interest in the use of indirect suggestion dates back to when he first began to study hypnosis in college. However, he waited until after receiving his doctoral degree to begin his formal research study with indirect and permissive hypnotic induction (Erickson, 1964/2001c, p. 1). As he continued to use indirect suggestion throughout his career, it provided the rationale behind his use of metaphor and stories (Matthews, Lankton, and Lankton, 1993), his multilevel use of language, and his skillful utilization of nonverbal communication.

Erickson believed that suggestion in psychotherapy should be indirect whenever possible (Erickson and Rossi, 1981). Some have mistaken this message as meaning that indirect suggestion is always more effective than direct suggestion, a notion that has been discredited in laboratory studies (Matthews, 2000). However, when considering Erickson's philosophy of healing, which includes the need for the practitioner to adapt therapy to the patient's theory of change, it becomes apparent why he would prefer indirect suggestion over direct suggestion. Indirect suggestions have a degree of ambiguity that allows greater freedom in responding (Matthews, Lankton, and Lankton, 1993).[2] Therefore, the effectiveness of indirect suggestion is not measured in terms of compliance with the practitioner's expectations but instead by the cumulative good that is accomplished in relation to the patient's needs.

Another reason for favoring indirect suggestion in certain instances is that this method of communication seems to reach parts of the mind that are not accessible by means of direct communication. These are the regions of the brain not mediated by

---

[1] The details of the above case report come in part from a conversation between Betty Alice Erickson and her mother, Elizabeth Erickson, many years after Erickson's death.

[2] Freedom of response, and thus increased satisfaction for subjectively experienced realities, is a very difficult thing to measure. This is especially true when using a standardized approach that relies on group averages for interpretation of results. Using the current tools of behavioral science, researchers are likely to produce results that favor the use of techniques that, unlike indirect suggestion, lend themselves to replication and prediction.

frontal-lobe activity. With every event, sensory stimuli travel through the brain using multiple pathways, thereby creating a multitude of implicit memories and expectations (Carlson, 2004). This physiology results in behaviors that the person sometimes cannot explain. It is these conditioned behaviors that often become the symptoms that bring people to therapy.

Rather than always attempting to make the unconscious conscious, Erickson would often deal with problems that existed outside the realm of conscious awareness using a form of communication that was also outside the realm of conscious awareness. Along these same lines, research has shown that affective priming (using classical conditioning) works better when the emotional primes are presented outside of conscious awareness (Murphy and Zajonc, 1993). If you want to help a person feel better about a certain stimulus, which makes them uncomfortable for reasons they cannot understand, then it is better to create a new positive association without evoking conscious awareness.

This style of communication is difficult to define. The term "indirect suggestion" has an implied meaning that covers nearly everything other than explicit commands. With both direct and indirect suggestion, ideas can be communicated through language, through nonverbal communication, or symbolic acts.[3] The difference is that with the use of indirect suggestion the desired outcome is not made explicit for conscious review. A direct suggestion ("Sit in the chair") is made indirect by use of implication ("After a while you might find that you grow tired of standing") or by asking a question ("Would you like to have a seat?") or by association ("My patients generally sit in that chair there") or by very broad statements of fact ("At some point, you're going to want to sit down"). Another method would be to say nothing while catching the client's gaze and then looking over at the empty chair. Yet another method would be to move the chair slightly toward the client with one's toe. The variety of ways to communicate something indirectly is virtually unlimited.

---

[3] For example, waving a white flag during a time of war is a symbolic act that results in direct communication.

The most common type of indirect suggestion is the implied directive. When Erickson found his son Robert injured and in pain, he told him, "That hurts awful bad! And it's going to keep on hurting for a little while." The implied directive was, "You can stop hurting in a little while." When one of Erickson's daughters returned from the orthodontist, and he commented, "That mouthful of hardware that you've got in your mouth is miserably uncomfortable and it's going to be a deuce of a job to get used to it," the implied directive was, "You *will* get used to it." A common element in each of these suggestions is the use of ideas in the opening of the statement that closely match the person's experience. This makes the rest of the suggestion more readily accepted (Erickson, 1976/2001).

Another good means of delivering an indirect suggestion is by asking a question. This is especially useful in hypnosis because it automatically focuses patients' attention inward, so that they can search for an answer. When you ask the patient, "How much time do *you* think will need to pass before you allow yourself to see your progress?" it produces a need to find an answer, so less energy is available to reject the suggestion that progress will be achieved. In addition to these types of remarks, Erickson would often ask questions that could not be answered entirely by conscious processes, "Would you like to go into trance now or in a few minutes?" It is evident that the answer to this question presupposes the idea that the patient will go into a trance (Erickson, 1976/2001). What is less evident is the larger implication: if healing is achieved by means of trance and the patient goes into a trance, then he is bound to heal.

Indirect suggestions can also be communicated by recognizing associations that patients automatically form and then using these associations as a sort of psychological "handle." It is a way of creating openings for meaningful dialogue without having to intrusively reach into someone else's psychological baggage. According to Erickson, the easiest way to help patients talk about their mothers is to talk about your own mother (Erickson, 1976/2001). After all, most of us remember from childhood how extraordinarily defensive a person can become if you are talking about *their* mother.

Along similar lines, if the practitioner wants to suggest to a woman who was abused sexually as a child the next step she should take in therapy, then this can be facilitated by making reference to a woman who was a patient and who had experienced sexual abuse, and who had made important gains in therapy by taking the next step. In this way, the suggestion is not imposed on the patient, who under such circumstances might experience needless performance anxiety: "The therapist has told me that I must take the next step, but what if I fail?" The use of indirect suggestion completely bypasses this sort of thing so that the client's response develops in a more spontaneous way.

Roxanna Klein remembers when she was very young running into the house one day to report that she had seen a "Kachina doll with wings." She was not old enough yet to recognize a dragonfly. She still remembers Erickson coming outside to investigate the situation and explaining to Roxanna that she had a very important talent in her way of finding precise words to express what she had seen. This was a direct suggestion that he continued to cultivate so that her positive association with certain words could later be used as indirect suggestion.

For example, as a child, Klein loved the taste and texture of stale bread. While happily watching her mother make bread pudding, she would ask her to set aside pieces of "tunchy" bread. Later, when Klein would worry over a school exam or meeting someone special the next day, Erickson would lovingly joke, "This is a problem that *tunchy* bread can resolve." The indirect suggestion was that the problem is a small one that can be met with humor and dealt with by reflecting on something that brings comfort. When Klein was pregnant, and worried about labor, Erickson told her that she should keep a slice of "tunchy" bread under her pillow, "so it will be ready any time you need it." She followed his recommendation, and it worked.

Another variation on indirect suggestion is the nonspecific use of inevitabilities. For instance, the direct suggestion, "Eventually, your eyes will close" is an inescapable suggestion. The only way to resist this suggestion is never to again sleep. The suggestion is made indirect by adding a nonspecific qualifier, "*Sooner or later* your eyes are going to close." For those not interested in achieving trance induction, the statement is easily modified: "Sooner or later you are going to see something about yourself that you have not noticed before." The advantage of mentioning an inevitable fact of life, in relation to the problem-solving endeavor, is that it helps focus the client's actions in a meaningful way. Whatever experience patients have in response to such suggestions is in a direction of therapeutic change (Erickson, 1976/2001).

The special advantage of using this form of suggestion is that it permits the practitioner to speak with absolute confidence, knowing that the patient is not being asked to do anything more or less than she has been doing for most of her life. "Sooner or later you will take a deep breath and find yourself feeling just a little bit more relaxed." The suggestion is inescapable. It is inevitable that this will occur, at least once, at some point in this person's future. As Erickson (1962/2001) explains, "Knowing then that [the practitioner] can reasonably and rightfully expect his patient to accomplish as much as thousands of other average patients have achieved, he can radiate full confidence and expectation to his patient as a nonverbal but highly effective communication which in turn will affect most favorably the effectiveness of the [therapy] technique" (p. 3). Of course, knowing Erickson, we understand that the success of the technique is not the primary objective. It is the communication of hope that provides the strongest basis for change.

In regard to the case of John and the two trees, one point that might be inferred is Erickson's desire to have John establish *some roots* in the Erickson home. He anticipated that his wife would survive him by many years. He clearly saw John as someone who would be a faithful friend to Mrs Erickson while she in turn afforded him purpose, meaning and connection to a loving family in his daily routine. Unfortunately, we do not have a full explanation of this case from Erickson. Both Mrs Erickson and Betty Alice Erickson know that he had an excellent eye for plants. He would have recognized early on that John's tree was not likely to thrive and intentionally maneuvered John into identifying with the stronger tree. But why did he turn this symbolic act into a competition? Erickson could have planted just one tree to suggest John's growth and connection to the family. One possible explanation is that Erickson was helping John develop his confidence in the way that a caring father helps boost his child's self-esteem. An example of this method is described in Chapter 12, in the case of a girl who was overwhelmed with feelings of failure at school (see p. 208). Erickson allowed her to win a bicycle race with him. This was an especially wonderful victory for the girl because she knew that her brother had already raced Erickson on a bicycle, and had lost! Whatever his reason for planting the two trees, it is clear that much of Erickson's foresight came from his passion for the growth of living things.

Permissive suggestion

Case report: The regulated diet

Erickson's help was requested by the parents of three seriously underweight children. The parents were putting a great deal of effort into the children's health. The mother explained to Erickson that she always had a perfectly balanced diet for them. Her nutritional regime was comprehensive and covered everything from each of the major food groups. She had the proper foods for breakfast, the proper foods for lunch, and the proper food for dinner. She wanted the children to achieve a healthy diet by conforming to her understanding of what they should eat, when they should eat it, and how they should eat it.

Erickson explained to the well-intentioned parents, "The problem is to teach the children to enjoy eating food." He felt the children must learn how to enjoy satisfying their hunger. Therefore Erickson made it clear to the parents that they should not try to force a specific diet on their children.

Erickson wanted the parents to tell their children that they would stop trying to interfere with their eating. The only requirement of the children was that they come to the table, at the appointed time, three times a day. The children were to be told that they could help themselves to whatever their mother placed on the table.

In order to meet the personality needs of the mother, Erickson told her, "You want a balanced diet. All right, let's go into training on this. Make a record of what Johnny eats. Make a record of what

Willie eats. And make a record of what Annie eats for each meal. At the end of the month add it up."

A month later, the mother came back and reported that the children had balanced their diets and gained weight. One of them started out and ate nothing but lettuce all day. On another day, he ate nothing but meat. On another day, he ate nothing but bread. As Erickson explains, "The children really went wild getting a sense of freedom." And, with this freedom came the opportunity to learn more about the dictates of their body's hunger.

(Erickson, 1958c)

"We are generally the better persuaded by the reasons we discover ourselves than by those given to us by others."
– Blaise Pascal, 1623–62

We see in Erickson's work a deep respect for the innate abilities of each individual. This is especially true in his conceptualization of permissive suggestion.

Although some use the terms "indirect" and "permissive" interchangeably, Erickson described permissive suggestion is an adaptation of indirect suggestion (Erickson, Hershman, and Sector, 1961, p. 272). The basic premise behind permissive suggestion is that people can be trusted to use their unconscious mind in order to discover the most appropriate solution for their problem.

When Erickson spoke of the "unconscious," he was referring to the ability of the mind to act as a storehouse of all that the person has seen, experienced, learned, and felt. He believed the unconscious should be identified as something that is essentially good, a protector and a helper, and that it can be called upon and trusted. As such, the patient's unconscious mind became one of Erickson's most important allies during treatment. He developed convincing methods for providing his patients with *permission* to access their hidden resources.

This is the background against which we make sense of permissive suggestion. The therapist must accept the idea that patients, with the exception of those who are severely mentally ill, will do the right thing for themselves, in the right sequence, and at the right time. In contrast to direct suggestion, Erickson used permissive suggestion to facilitate new learning by allowing patients to *create their own solutions* in their own way (Rossi, 1973). In this way, patients learn to trust what will be discovered within themselves during the process of therapy.

This approach has definite advantages over other means of suggestion. Research from social psychology has shown that when patients attribute therapeutic change to internal factors such as personality change or new coping skills, *the change tends to be long-term*. Alternatively, if patients attribute therapeutic change to external factors such as the therapist or his interventions, the change tends to be short-lived. The locus of attribution, either internal or external, appears to set up self-fulfilling prophecies (Weinberger, 1994, 1995). Permissive suggestion allows patients to act not only as an essential collaborator in the therapy process but also as the one who has the final say in how they conduct themselves in the future.

Although it is classified here as a single technique, there are many ways of achieving permissive suggestion. What these have in common is the use of ambiguous stimuli designed to elicit responses based upon experiential learnings (Erickson, 1958). This encourages patients to develop their own subjectively meaningful conclusions rather than be told what to think or do. The ambiguity in suggestions and stories stimulates mental activity and enhances communication. It is not limited to the practice of hypnosis (Lankton, 2001/2003, p. 8). Similar to the concept of gardening, Erickson would often plant seeds, in the form of new ideas, and then wait to see what would grow.

One means of providing a permissive suggestion is to frame each injunction as an option rather than a command. For instance, when the suggestion for hand levitation is framed as a mere suggestion—"Your hand *might* begin to feel lighter, *maybe* in the fingertips, *maybe* just a tingling on the palm, I don't know but you can notice a difference in your hands"—then there is an opportunity for the patient to decide what the hand will actually do.

The same effect is achieved by using the word "perhaps." For example, *"Perhaps* this might be the time to recall a long-forgotten memory that is important to you." This qualifying term frames the idea as a suggestion rather than an order. So there is no need for the patient to struggle against an external force.

Yet another means of focusing attention on opportunities is by pointing out the patient's autonomy in relation to a specific behavior. As Erickson might say, "I do not know whether or not you are going into a trance as you have asked" (Erickson, 1964/2001b, p. 3). This defines this situation as one in which it is clear that the patient is in charge of his destiny. Erickson had no way to know if what the patient had asked for would occur. He merely suggested that it would.

A second means of achieving permissive suggestion is by use of generalities. As Erickson explains, "You make general statements that a person can apply to specifics within his own life" (Erickson, 1973/2001a, p. 2). This is surprisingly easy to do. Most of us went to school, learned to read and write, played with friends, loved a pet, wished to be loved by our parents etc. When a general statement is made, with specifics only about peripheral details, the patient tends to fill in the rest with personally meaningful facts. "Your first day of school was an important accomplishment. And everything in the schoolyard seemed so much larger to you on the first day, but it did not seem so much so on your last day of school. And there were other feelings that changed inside of you, some of which you may not have thought of for many, many years." With this type of suggestion there is greater freedom for patients to explore their unique life experiences and apply them to the current situation.

A third means of achieving permissive suggestion is by using open-ended statements that suggest many possible options of response (Erickson, 1976/2001). For example, "Every person has abilities not known to the self. There are memories, thoughts, feelings, and sensations completely or partially forgotten by the conscious mind that are available to the unconscious and can be experienced whenever the unconscious is ready." With the use of open-ended suggestion, whatever the subject experiences in response to the stimuli is a valid response that serves as a foundation for future work (Erickson, 1976/2001, pp. 4–22). The open-ended suggestion permits patients to select experiences that are most appropriate for their unique needs.

If you think back to the case at the beginning of this section, it should be clear by now that the children's need to discover their own appetites is analogous to most every patient's need to discover what is required from therapy. This is the spirit of permissive suggestion. Therapeutic nourishment is not shoved down people's throats but is instead spread out as a feast from which patients can select what best suits their needs. It is a buffet table from which the patient can choose all or nothing, old favorites, or something new. As Erickson explained about the children's appetites, it is not helpful to impose upon them something that should be experienced as an opportunity.

Interspersal and repetition

Case report: The man with phantom-limb pain

A man in his late sixties underwent a hemipelvectomy following the discovery of a cancerous tumor. After the removal of his leg he developed phantom limb pain. The pain was experienced as a feeling of his toes being severely twisted, his foot being bent double, and his leg being twisted and pulled far back behind him. It came in convulsive episodes throughout the day and night, causing him to be covered in perspiration, to sometimes fall to the floor, and to experience involuntary outcries. Between these severe episodes there was a constant aching pain. The man had endured his condition for the past six years, during which he became highly dependent on Demerol injections, sometimes as much as 100mg, 12–16 times in a 24-hour period. He was absolutely desperate for relief and explained to Erickson that he did not want to live life as a dope addict: "I've seen them all around the world. I am a man, not a freak! I don't want to be torn to pieces by pain and drugs. But I can't last much longer. So do something, anything your conscience allows!"

The man had already experienced several failures with hypnosis. He repeatedly apologized to Erickson: "I am a lousy, impossible subject. But I can't help being bossy, stubborn, constantly watchful, and disputatious." Direct hypnosis would not work with him. As the patient explained, "Any help you give me for my pain and my drug addition you'll have to sneak in when I am not looking. I've been top-dog so long I can't stop even when it's for my own good."

Despite these obstacles, the patient knew other professionals respected Erickson's work and was hopeful that this doctor could help him, "Dr von Dedenroth … described you as having a hypnotic technique so sneaky that you could keep dry in a heavy rain, and the way he said that, I believed him. So you've got my permission to do anything you can get by with."

Erickson engaged the man in casual conversation and discovered he was gregarious and charming. He had dropped out of high school and educated himself through extensive reading. He owned seven business corporations, having progressed from a childhood of extreme poverty to great wealth. He had endowed orphanages, hospitals, libraries, and museums. He had traveled extensively throughout the northern hemisphere. He was always intensely interested in the personal lives of others. As he explained, "I have never met anybody I didn't like, including scoundrels." However, in all of this conversation he never related any of his personal experiences, other than the experience of pain.

Erickson spent the first two sessions, a total of six hours, distracting the man with casual conversation, interspersed with suggestions for trance behavior. Erickson did not attempt any suggestion for pain relief until the third session, when the man demonstrated an ability to experience amnesia for everything discussed during trance. Under these conditions the man obeyed instructions without question.

Erickson used the hypnotic sessions to discuss in great detail all of the things that he knew would be most interesting and absorbing for this person. Throughout the narrative he interspersed suggestions for relief from pain and freedom from addiction. These themes were repeated, again and again but in different contexts. Afterwards, these trances were consciously recognized by the man merely as unaccountable lapses of time.

Following several sessions, the man became suspicious of his conversations with Erickson: "I don't know what you are doing, but my problems are decreasing." Erickson would not admit to succeeding with hypnosis but instead evaded the topic: "Maybe I won't have to do anything." Eventually, the issue of using hypnosis to help his pain was dropped altogether. When Erickson did mention hypnosis it was in relation to other patients. While discussing this and a variety of other topics, Erickson continued to intersperse suggestions of pain control within the conversation.

After two months, the patient declared he needed no further help. Nine months later, he returned to Erickson following a severe attack of Hong Kong influenza and the near death of his adored wife from the same illness. In response to extreme stress, his pain and drug dependency recurred. As he explained to Erickson, "I do not know how in hell you talk me out of pain and Demerol, but you sure do, and that damn flu has put me right back to where I was when I first came, maybe worse."

Erickson again used the same technique, making no effort to use hypnosis during the first two sessions. This was discouraging for the man: "I'll try another couple of sessions, and when they peter out, I'll take your advice about using some other drug than this damn Demerol." At the close of the third session, he aroused from a deep trance without knowing he had been in a trance. Suddenly he became startled, looked at his watch, recognized that three hours had passed, then exclaimed, "You son of a bitch. You sneaked past me again, when I wasn't looking!" Erickson had recognized that the patient was likely to reject his suggestions had he moved too quickly.

There was a second recurrence of intense pain, over a year later, following surgery for an enlarged prostate gland. During his hospitalization he received help from Erickson by phone. When he was released from the hospital, he came to Phoenix for a more satisfactory re-establishment of his pain relief and freedom from drug dependency.

(Erickson, 1973/2001b, pp. 10–14)

Further into therapy, Erickson decided it would be helpful for the man to watch someone who was skillful at self-hypnosis. He brought in Betty Alice, who remembers using arm catalepsy for her induction, as usual, but then hallucinating her hand still on her leg. This resulted in two right hands, either of which could disappear and reappear. In this state of confusion, Betty Alice experienced anesthesia in both the real and hallucinated arm, without regard to the physical reality of either. Completely absorbed in her trance, she turned to the man. "Do you know which hand is real and which is not?" she asked. He said he did and Betty Alice asked him how. "One I can see. And the other I can't." Betty Alice replied, "I can see them both. I know one isn't real. But I do not know which one." Erickson then asked the man, "How can Betty Alice determine the difference between the one that is real and the one that is not?" The man thought about his own experiences and the nature of the sensations coming from a real leg and a phantom limb.

Although he was obviously pleased with his therapy, the man never did lose his phantom-limb pain completely. The recurrences he said were, "nothing like the real thing, but bad enough to worry me. I just have to take a little time out, knowing that I can do without them."

(Erickson, 1973/2001b, p. 14)

When studying hypnosis, it is apparent that the technique of repeating ideas, to increase their influence, has been practiced since suggestion was first identified as a fundamental strategy. But even before its use in hypnosis, repetition has been practiced by medicine men and witch doctors in the form of ritual and chants.

When Western missionaries began entering remote jungle villages, where the witch doctor was the spiritual authority, a clash of cultures was not only inevitable but sometimes deadly. This conflict was resolved peacefully in one particular instance when two Christian missionaries agreed to a public competition to determine whose magic was more powerful. At the appointed time, the missionaries were instructed by the witch doctor to simply hold his staff and keep it from lifting off the ground. They were encircled by the villagers who followed the witch doctor in a repetitious chant: "The pole must rise … The pole must rise … The pole must rise!" Drums were beaten in time with the chant and, after a period of unrelenting suggestion, the missionaries' muscles began to tighten. Shortly thereafter, beads of perspiration ran down their face as the pole slowly lifted from the ground. Having proved his point, the witch doctor was then willing to allow the missionaries to enter into his village. Assuming the missionaries did not fabricate this story, which is not likely since it was a source of shame, it is interesting to speculate on what would have happened if they had simply loosened their grip. Those readers who understand the arm-levitation technique will recognize the witch doctor's method as a simple variation of a challenge suggestion—"*the pole levitation technique.*"

When we consider the amount of skill or training required to successfully use suggestion, it is interesting to think back to innocent childhood games, such as "Light as a feather, stiff as a board." Many a child has delighted in watching their friends stiffen up in response to the chant and then seem to float into the air as the others effortlessly lift the stiffened body using only one finger each. The power of repeated suggestion is not a strange or uncommon phenomenon. When people hear something repeated enough times, they eventually begin to believe it.

When suggestion is used for clinical purposes, there are one or more helpful ideas that are targeted for communication to the patient. However, just as medicinal drugs must be accepted by the physiology of the body, in order to do any good, therapeutic ideas require psychological acceptance. The technique of repetition appears to be helpful in this regard. It is easier to reject unfamiliar ideas than those to which we have grown accustomed. Along these lines, research has shown that presenting the same object to people on multiple occasions (mere exposure) will increase the liking for the object (Bornstein, 1989; Zajonc and Markus, 1982). Confidently presenting the same idea, repetitiously, can sometimes produce greater movement toward its realization.

When we consider the importance of acceptance during the use of suggestion, it becomes apparent that it is not helpful to antagonize the patient with monotonous redundancies. Erickson's solution for this was to expand the technique of repetition by interspersing his suggestions throughout an ongoing dialogue. When an idea is communicated as a brief statement, it is not as likely to arouse critical review. As the basic suggestion is continually revisited, throughout the conversation, it becomes more and more familiar and is thereby absorbed into the patient's thinking. This is the essence of Erickson's interspersal technique (Erickson, 1966/2001).

When considering the case of the man with the phantom-limb pain, the use of suggestion by means of interspersal technique is apparent in each session. What is less obvious is Erickson's use of repetition at the macro level. A year later, when the man returned for therapy, Erickson repeated his procedure precisely, first waiting two sessions before attempting therapy, then offering suggestion for pain relief at the end of third. And again the man responded with the same astonished behavior he had learned one year previous.

When seeking to learn more about hypnosis, Betty Alice asked Erickson about his reasons for her demonstration. Erickson explained that the man was having difficulty interpreting the sensations that his nerves were sending. By default, the signals were interpreted as pain. While watching Betty Alice hallucinate a pseudo-arm, the man was likely to reference his bodily pseudo-sensations in order to make sense of her comments. Therefore, anything he said to her would at some level be connected to his problem of phantom-limb pain. The man was then given the task of helping her understand the subtle differences between real sensations and those that are "hallucinated." By using her as a model, Erickson was teaching the man how to experience dissociation in relation to a limb *that in reality did not exist*. Using this absorbing double-dissociation, Erickson helped the man refine his ability to interpret these signals. In order to comply with Erickson's request, the man first had to dissociate from immediate sensations in his body, and then had to speculate on sensations in an arm that not only did not belong to him but that also did not exist! The problem he was given was parallel to his. As the saying goes, "It is always easier to see solutions when the problems belong to others."

When there was a great deal of resistance, Erickson often used distraction along with suggestion. While describing this case, Erickson explains that the interspersing of therapeutic suggestions among suggestions for trance maintenance will often make the therapeutic suggestions more effective. The therapeutic suggestions are heard and understood, but before the patient can take issue with them, their attention is captured by the trance-maintenance suggestions (Erickson, 1973/2001b). If the patient does in fact maintain the trance behavior, then both sets of suggestions are simultaneously ratified at an unconscious level, "If I am still in trance, as suggested, then the suggestions given to me during trance must be working!"

When using hypnosis in therapy, the trance induction and trance maintenance represent, in microcosm, the success of therapy as a whole. With the successful induction of trance, a hopeful situation is created: "This person can get me into a trance, when no one else could, therefore he must be capable of providing the help I need." With this in mind, it is easy to see why it would be meaningful for Erickson to use repeated trance sessions for those, such as this man, who need a great deal of reassurance.

When the time is right, one can find hope even within the context of disturbing realities. Successful healing is not the same as magic. Erickson never did cure the man of the phantom-limb pain. Instead he helped transform the experience into something that he could *live* with. This allowed the man to experience many more years of happy living. *With time,* the cancer found its way back into his body. The pain was especially bad and the prognosis poor. When faced with the prospect of spending the rest of his life doped up on drugs and in a state of constant *physical deterioration,* the man chose a different alternative: he shot himself.

The confusion technique

Case report: The woman who felt she could not be hypnotized

A woman entered Erickson's office for her first appointment in what appeared to be a state of extreme ambivalence. Erickson interpreted her behavior as being simultaneously halting and uncertain, yet she walked into the office with a forceful and defiant stride. She sat down in her chair in a rigid position with the palms of her hands braced against her knees. She introduced herself by describing the failure of her previous doctors who had spent as many as thirty hours attempting unsuccessfully to hypnotize her. She then added, "All of them told me that I was too resistant to be hypnotized, but they all said you could do it. But I went to the other two because they were near my home town. I didn't want to come all the way to Phoenix to be hypnotized. But even my family doctor has told me it would help overcome my resistances to therapy."

Erickson recognized that although she could not make sense of her need to both approach and avoid therapy, she was earnestly seeking help. After hearing her explain in detail how the other doctors had failed to hypnotize her, Erickson felt she would attempt to embroil him in a contest instead of accepting therapy. So he brusquely responded, "Well, let's get this clear. Three doctors, all good men, just as good as I am, have worked hard and long on you. They found you to be too resistant, as I will too. So let's have that understood at once."

Erickson then altered his voice inflection and tempo as he declared, "*I can't hypnotize you*, justyourarm."

In a bewildered fashion she replied, "Can't hypnotize me, just my arm ... I don't understand what you mean." Erickson repeated himself with slow, heavy emphasis, "*That's exactly what I mean. I can't hypnotize you.*" Then, with a soft, gentle voice he added, "Justyourarm ... see." As he spoke the word "see," Erickson gently touched her hand so that it would lift in an upward movement. He slowly withdrew his fingers and her hand remained cataleptically suspended in midair.

As she watched her arm caught in this unexpected position, Erickson softly intoned, "Just close your eyes, take a deep breath, so deeply asleep, and as you do so, your left hand will slowly come to rest on your thigh and remain there continuously as you sleep deeply and comfortably until I tell you to awaken." Within five minutes after her entrance into the office she was in a deep, somnambulistic trance.

(Erickson, 1964/2001d, p. 30)

The confusion technique is an advanced technique, of which Erickson was the master. Although the use of confusion is more accurately viewed as a step toward increased responsiveness, rather than suggestion proper, its significant role in Erickson's method of interpersonal influence warrants mention in this section. He used confusion to prepare patients for change. Confusion was often incorporated during hypnotic induction to foster a state of greater receptivity. As can be seen in the example, just a little bit of confusion is sometimes enough to shift a person into an entirely new mindset.

Confusion is often a byproduct of the unexpected. As Erickson explains, "Whenever you do the unexpected you jog a person out of their setting" (Erickson and Rossi, 1976, p. 154). Betty Alice Erickson recalls a foster child who had difficulty adjusting to her new parents. This family consulted with Erickson for quite some time, and the mother became a friend of Betty Alice Erickson. The young girl, Sara, was extremely controlling and restricted her own behavior in many unhealthy ways. The mother complained, "Sara doesn't have anything else to do all day except exactly what she wants to do—she doesn't have to go to work or fix dinner or pick up her sisters from school. She can take forever to eat her breakfast or brush her teeth because she has no schedule she must maintain." Much of her defiance was passive resistance.

Sara was frantically searching for security and did not feel safe unless she was controlling others. The momentary relief she experienced, while in control, produced a strong secondary gain. However, by making things so difficult for the family she had little opportunity to believe that she was truly a welcome addition to the family. Direct confrontation and ordinary punishments did not curb the behaviors, since she merely became more insecure. This self-perpetuating cycle was nearly impossible to escape.

Erickson intervened by instructing the mother to make certain that routines in the home were varied in unexpected but enjoyable ways. It was essential that the unexpected activities involve the rest of the family. He explained that, if Sara participated, her parents were setting the standards. If she didn't, everyone else was simply enjoying new and exciting behaviors that she had no reason to reject, thereby building her desire to eventually become a part of the family.

The parents followed Erickson's advice. For example, the family had an "upside-down night:" everyone went to bed with their head at the foot of the bed, with their feet resting on a pillow. The brother and two young sisters were delighted by the silly game. Another day, the mother organized a swim party and included several neighbor children. Everyone was to swim in their socks, including Mom. The children were further delighted when the mother told them that lunch would be "backwards." Everybody got to eat dessert before the sandwich, which was a "bread sandwich"—a slice of bread sandwiched between two slices of bologna. Sara was upset because this was not how it was "supposed to be." The mother's behavior was confusing. However, Sara decided to join the group and thereby accept her mother's definition of how swimming and lunch would be. Because of the way the situation had been structured, Sara had fun while submitting to her mother's authority, something that added yet another level of confusion.

Confusion in its most potent form is derived from the *uncertain behavior of the patient* in response to the unexpected action of the therapist. As explained by Erickson:

> The Confusion Technique is a presentation of ideas and understandings conducive of mental activity and response but so intermingled with seemingly related, valid but actually nonpertinent communications that responses are inhibited, frustration and uncertainty of mind engendered. The culmination occurs in a final suggestion permitting a ready and easy response satisfying to the subjects and validated by each subject's own ... experiential learnings.

> (Erickson, 1964/2001d, p. 32)

Erickson would often achieve this unique experience of confusion through the use of arm levitation. In most cases, subjects of the technique were utterly confused by the behavior of their own limb as it remained cataleptic in the air. For Erickson, this type of confusion constituted a special form of humor (Erickson, 1964/ 2001d), something that patients could be amused by and enjoy.

Erickson's playful use of confusion is evident from the moment when he first recognized its potential as an important hypnotic technique. The incident occurred on a windy day in 1923. As a young college student, Erickson was rushing to attend the first collegiate seminar on hypnosis conducted in the United States. Unexpectedly, a man came around the corner of a building and the two collided. Before the man could recover his poise, Erickson glanced at his watch and courteously stated, "It's exactly 10 minutes of two." In reality, it was closer to 4 p.m. Erickson then walked on. About a half a block away he turned and saw the man still staring at him, bewildered by the remark. This was not the first time Erickson had playfully initiated this sort of confusion. However, it was after this event that he recognized the potential of the technique to create a "feeling of mental eagerness on their part for some comprehensible understanding" (Erickson, 1964/2001d, p. 2).

In order to be as clear as possible about confusion, it is helpful to recognize the variety of ways in which it can be created. These include the use of irrelevancy, non sequitur, a play on the double meaning of words, the overelaboration of detail, offering a series of contradictory suggestions, and the sudden interruption of well-established behavioral patterns. The last of these was famously applied by Erickson as part of his handshake induction.

The handshake induction was used by Erickson in many of his teaching demonstrations to demonstrate just how quickly a state of deep inner absorption can be achieved. The demonstration subject would hardly have stepped onto the stage before finding himself in a deep trance. In order to ensure a successful demonstration, Erickson would sometimes pick his subjects by observing their behavior before the lecture as he went around the room shaking hands, using a lingering grip. This would allow him to estimate which person in the audience would respond most readily to this type of induction. Once the person was called to the stage, Erickson would extend his hand, but then suddenly interrupt the automatic movement of the other person's arm by taking the subject's hand and placing it cataleptically in front of the subject's face. The confusion created by this technique comes not only from Erickson's unexpected behavior but also from the person not knowing what to do with his or her own hand. Following this sort of procedure, the person would be fully absorbed in the process of cooperating with subsequent suggestions from Erickson (Erickson, 1961a, 1961b).

In the examples mentioned thus far, it is the unexpected experience of arm levitation that serves as the basis for the confusion. An interesting question to ask is would the same technique work as well with someone who is already trained in hypnosis and experienced with arm levitation. As an experiment, Short conducted a demonstration during which a volunteer, from an audience of practiced hypnotic operators, was instructed to do everything in his power to resist hypnosis. After asking some preliminary questions about his confidence in his ability to resist suggestion, the subject was asked if it would be all right to touch him on his *right* hand, as a cue for arm levitation. After he agreed, Short then carelessly reached for his left hand. In order to correct the situation, the subject spontaneously lifted his right hand into the air. At the same instant, Short withdrew his hand and stared intently at the subject's right hand. This combined action left his hand with no place to go, therefore it remained frozen in a cataleptic state. The subject was then told to close his eyes and go into a deep trance. This resulted in a somnambulistic trance that permitted the demonstration of several advanced hypnotic phenomena. Similar to the handshake induction, this subject expected the arm levitation to be conducted in a certain way. It was his confusion over the unexpected behavior and the interruption of his practiced patterns of behavior that prepared the way for the demonstration.

Confusion can also be introduced through verbal means alone. A verbal confusion technique commonly used by Erickson was to tell irrelevant stories and make non sequitur remarks (Erickson and Rossi, 1981, p. 166). These are otherwise sensible statements that find their way into a line of reasoning to which they do not belong. This is a natural behavior that can be observed in everyday events. When a non sequitur occurs within the context of a single statement, the results are often humorous. For instance, a person who was familiar with a certain bistro warned his friends, "Nobody sits in that part of the restaurant anymore: it's too crowded." As a standalone comment, the statement is amusing. But, when a series of non sequiturs begin to obscure the meaning of an important conversation, then the frustrated attempts to understand what is being communicated results in an intensified desire to latch onto some idea that can be readily understood. Similar to the practice of lowering one's voice to a whisper while making an important point, this verbal confusion technique is a method of *capturing* the listener's full *attention*, with the added advantage of motivating the listener to put energy into *understanding* the ideas that have been communicated.

The confusion technique can also be based upon a play on words. The more practiced and clear clinicians are in making their confounded statements, the more likely their success in capturing the subject's attention. In some instances, Erickson used a play on words to confuse the patient's orientation to time:

> For example, one may declare so easily that the present and the past can be so readily summarized by the simple statement, "That which now *is* will soon be, *was* yesterday's *future* even as it *will* be tomorrow's *was*." Thus are the past, the present, and the future all used in reference to the reality of "today."

> (Erickson, 1964/2001d, p. 30)

Similarly, Erickson would also use elaboration and repetition of modifiers in order to confuse the patient's orientation to space. One such technique was called "here, there, this, and that." When he had patients who were resistant to the therapy they were seeking, Erickson would offer a casual comment that might sound something like this, "While sitting in *that* chair you are resistant. But would you have been resistant had you sat in *this* other chair? Or would you be nonresistant in *this* chair and thus leave your resistances in *that* chair you now occupy?" In some instances he might point toward a nonexistent chair, which was then automatically hallucinated.

While making these statements Erickson would speak in a deliberate manner with emphasis added through proper inflection. Without leaving enough time for the patient to take issue with what has just been said, Erickson would add, "You can mentally consider changing chairs and sitting *here* in this one and leaving resistance in that chair *there* or sitting in *that* chair *there* while your resistance remains *here* in this chair *here*. You might also try sitting in *that* other chair there without resistance and then coming back *here* to this chair *here* and taking up your resistances either to keep or to leave them *there* in *this* or *that* chair or *here* or *there*." Erickson would continue to elaborate on *here*, *there*, *this*, and *that* with as much varied repetition as necessary to achieve a sufficient state of confusion (Erickson, 1964/2001d).

It is important to recognize that in the example above the *confusion is tied to the patient's resistances*, thus they are given the opportunity to do away with both the confusion and resistances as soon as they begin to cooperate with the therapy. In contrast, *the actual content of therapy should be stated very clearly and simply*. Having been aroused into greater and greater effort to develop new under-standings, the subject is properly rewarded with a clear-cut defin-itive statement that can be readily seized upon. Even with the supplemental use of confusion, the general rule for suggestion is *the simpler the better*.

It is important to recognize that the confusion technique was developed by Erickson for use with a certain type of patient. According to him, "It is best employed with highly intelligent sub-jects interested in the hypnotic process, or with those consciously unwilling to go into a trance despite an unconscious willingness" (Erickson, 1958g, p. 98). It is not appropriate to use verbal confusion with a patient who is already highly responsive with sufficient motivation to consider whatever ideas that clinician has to offer.

One last point to consider is the role of confusion in the practice of psychotherapy as a whole. Later in his career, Erickson went as far as to say, "It [confusion] is the basis of all good techniques" (Erickson, Rossi, and Rossi, 1976, p. 107). This is a broad claim for the role of confusion. Erickson's line of reasoning is best under-stood from a learning perspective. Most will agree that, as long as a person maintains a sense of perfect comprehension, there is no need to assimilate new information. Rather than using the term *confusion*, Jean Piaget (1896–1980) speaks of *disequilibrium* as a pre-requisite for exploratory learning. From Piaget's perspective, it is only when assimilation will not work that accommodation to new realities becomes necessary. This growth-promoting view of dis-equilibrium fits with the therapeutic foundations of learning from which Erickson worked. If he was primarily interested in the re-education of the patient (see p. 23), then some amount of con-fusion would be necessary.

As for the case cited at the beginning of this section, what exactly happened? The woman had gone to a great deal of trouble in seek-ing therapy. She was desperate for help, enough so to leave her hometown and travel to Phoenix for treatment. But all of her past learning experiences with hypnosis had really built up the belief that she would not respond to therapeutic suggestion. Any con-ventional use of suggestion that she could recognize and under-stand was doomed to failure. Guided by these expectations, she was compelled to agree with Erickson when he said, "I can't hyp-notize you." And, while she was still in this accepting frame of mind, he quickly added, "*just your arm.*" This was confusing and therefore difficult to refute. She could not negate his assertion because he had clearly stated the thing that she had come to Phoenix to prove. So there was no longer any need to resist. But the last three words created enough inner disequilibrium that she was forced to ask for some explanation. While complying with her request for clarification, Erickson added a second command, "*See!*" When Erickson touched her hand, an automatic movement was activated. Since childhood she had learned that, if someone touches your hand, you must respond with some sort of move-ment. Now she could "see" her arm behaving in a way she could not understand. By this time, the situation had been transformed from a contest between two people to one of joint cooperation and participation in the shared task of achieving the therapeutic goal (Erickson, 1964/2001d).

The general application of suggestion

"The whole doctrine of animal magnetism can thus be summed up in two words: believe and want. I believe I have the power to act on the vital principle in all humans. I want to make use of this power for their benefit. If you also believe and want, you can do as much as I."
– Marquis de Puységur, 1787

Although he was well practiced in the formal induction rituals used by traditional hypnotists, Erickson believed that the *agency of suggestion is best achieved within the context of a flexible, cooperative interpersonal relationship*. While offering therapeutic suggestions, Erickson crafted his remarks using various direct, indirect, and permissive suggestions intended to channel patients' reactions into receptive and responsive behavior (Erickson, 1964/2001b). All of these served the general purpose of building a relationship in which patients could discover unrealized resources and potential for healing. Similarly, modern researchers have begun to recognize the importance of forming a cooperative interpersonal relationship noting that positive alliance is one of the best predictors of therapeutic outcome (Horvath & Symonds, 1991) and that in therapy, alliance accounts for as much as 54% of the total variance (Wampold, 2001).

Erickson's masterful use of suggestion was extraordinarily diverse and therefore difficult to cover in one brief chapter. Fortunately, his approach to hypnosis has been well documented and thoroughly analyzed in many other sources (e.g. Battino and South, 2005; Erickson, Rossi, and Rossi, 1976; Erickson and Rossi, 1979; Erickson and Rossi, 1981; Gilligan, 1987; Gordon and Myers-Anderson, 1981; Lankton and Lankton, 1983, Zeig, 1980).

At this time, there is no question that suggestion can have a dramatic impact on volitional behavior and physiological functioning. Over one hundred years of research supports this notion. The strategy of suggestion, whether in the form of hypnosis, placebo therapy, or indirect suggestion, is particularly effective with refractory disorders or those that have a strong psychosomatic component. It is with this group of problems that the use of suggestion will have seemingly miraculous results. The use of suggestion is also appropriate as an adjunct therapy for other psychological and/or biological problems.

When it comes to a determination of which techniques produce the best results, there is not a clear consensus. A review of the history of magnetism and hypnosis makes clear the fact that each pioneer has had his own favored technique and, for that person, this technique has worked more effectively than all others. For Anton Mesmer (1734–79) it was use of a conduit containing magnetic fluid; for the Marquis de Puységur (1751–1825) is was stroking areas of the body such as the solar plexus and the eyes; for Jean Martin Charcot (1825–93) there were hysterogenic zones on the body that produced four stages of hysteria; for James Braid (1795–1859) it was the act of staring at a shiny object; for Émile Coué (1857–1926) it was the daily recitation of the autosuggestion formula, "Every day in every way I'm getting better and better." But, when we come to Erickson, it is more difficult to pin him down to a single technique. He seemed willing to use whatever worked, whether verbal, nonverbal, or symbolic. With Erickson there seemed to be a greater appreciation for the essence of the strategy underlying any given technique.

When modern standardized research is applied to control for experimenter bias, the differences between hypnotic techniques seem to disappear. For instance, an overview of research that seeks to compare the effectiveness of suggestion following hypnotic induction and direct suggestion without induction (also known as waking suggestion) indicates that the results are generally equivalent (Short, 1999). As others have attempted to compare the use of direct suggestion with indirect suggestion, the results are mixed. In some instances direct suggestion seems to be more effective in producing measurable results while in others indirect suggestion is found to be more favorable (Matthews, Lankton, and Lankton, 1993). In fact, the same finding has been generalized to the field of therapy as a whole. Often referred to as the "Dodo bird verdict," the clear consensus among therapy outcome researchers is that the differences between types of treatment are not significant (Kirsch, 1990). Instead, it is the quality of the client's participation in therapy that stands out as the most important determinant of outcome (Orlinsky, Grawe, and Parks, 1994; Orlinsky, Rønnestad, and Willutzki, 2004).

When stepping back from the intellectual boxes created by a given theoretical orientation, one sees that the long and highly successful history of clinical suggestion demonstrates that the specifics of technique are not as important as the therapist's confidence that a patient can and will respond to suggestion.

In a landmark study, Lerner and Fiske (1973) found *that the therapist's belief that he or she could help was a better predictor of outcome than patient attributes* that previously have been claimed to predict outcome. Just as illuminating is Rosenthal's groundbreaking study in which teacher's expectations for student success were identified as having a significant impact on school performance. The most shocking finding in this study was that, as a result of self-fulfilling prophecy, students in the high-performance group showed a significant change in pre- and post-measure of intellectual ability (Rosenthal and Jacobson, 1968). Here we see that it is not the technique that matters as much as the ideas that are communicated to the client.

Six years prior to Rosenthal's discovery, while clarifying his position on the essence of hypnotic induction, Erickson emphatically declared:

> Every doctor needs ... an intense feeling of, "This I can do. And this other I can have done. And all the rest, if there is any more, lies in the hands of fate aided by all the good that I can do." ... To induce a trance, one needs to communicate by words, bearing, manner, emotional attitude, intellectual awareness that the patient is really and truly expected, confidently expected, to be as able to learn how to develop a trance as readily and as well as any of his fellows.

(Erickson, 1962/2001, pp. 1–3)

From this chapter's detailed discussion of suggestion there are some general points that apply to most of therapy. Like it or not, the effect of suggestion does not disappear just because the practitioner does not plan to use hypnosis. This fact creates a certain set of responsibilities. In best practice, all therapists should consider the benefits of enthusiastically explaining to their patients the known benefits of treatment. However, if this communication is producing a paradoxical effect, then it may be necessary to express doubt in the usefulness of therapy. It is often helpful to explain in detail why the patient is likely to benefit from treatment. However, if the patient has a history of self-sabotage, then it may be better to distract the client from the actual process of therapy. Typically, therapists should make certain that the processes of therapy are experienced as "doable" by the patient and provide some means of allowing patients to see their progress. However, there are undoubtedly exceptions to this rule as well. The major point is the importance of *watching* to see what effect a particular suggestion is having and then altering one's methods accordingly. Therapy is offered as a bridge that allows the client to cross from a position of distress to recognition of what can be done. This is the type of suggestion that transforms despair into hope.

Chapter 11

Reorientation

This chapter provides a means of conceptualizing one of the most pervasive strategies in all of psychotherapy. Reorientation can be seen underlying a wide variety of highly effective techniques used by Erickson and others. Because these strategies are not mutually exclusive, varying degrees of reorientation can be seen in each of the strategies listed in this book. However, in this chapter special emphasis is placed on techniques that are best explained as a method of providing the patient with a new perspective. As will be seen in the following case reports, reorientation may involve a single statement yet the effect can be life changing.

Case report: The woman who hid her beauty

A college girl came to Erickson for help with obesity. She was about 100 pounds over weight. While explaining the problem to Erickson she summed up her opinion of herself by stating, "I am just a fat slob." Looking at the disagreeable expression on her face and listening to her unhappy tone of voice, Erickson decided that she was experiencing a great deal of misery and emotional turmoil. In this unhappy state of mind the only ideas she would be willing to hear were those that matched her frame of reference. As Erickson explained, "I recognized that I could not give her any unpleasant ideas about her body that she did not already have." So he told her, "I really don't believe you know how disagreeable your fatness is to you. So tonight, before you go to bed, get in the nude, stand in front of a full-length mirror and really see how much you dislike all of that fat you have." These statements captured the girl's attention. The assignment was something which she knew that she could do. She was well practiced at being self-critical.

Then Erickson added, "And if you really think hard enough, and look through that layer of blubber that you have got wrapped around you, you will see a very pretty feminine figure. But it is buried rather deeply." After giving her some time to deal with these new positive ideas about herself, Erickson placed her in control of her therapy by asking, "What do you think you ought to do to get that figure excavated?" She was able to come up with her own solution. It apparently worked for her. As Erickson reports, "She began excavating it at about five pounds a week."

(Erickson, 1965b)

The concept of learned helplessness is a familiar idea coming from research done years ago in which a lab animal was conditioned to lie helplessly while receiving shocks from an electric grid, even though escape was readily available. This behavioral outcome has been used as a model for understanding situational depression. The idea is that a child who is not allowed to escape painful outcomes will eventually be conditioned to respond to any stressor with withdrawal and self-devaluation.

The concept of learned helplessness even has implications for understanding resiliency. In all instances of psychological dysfunction a person's readiness to move out of a state of distress is limited by a conceptual understanding of what is possible. In other words, when a person can see no way out, the energy for improvement is lost and there is no resiliency. But what happens when a new view of the situation is produced? When circumstances are viewed in a new way, new options are recognized. As with all of the other strategies, reorientation is a proven tactic that has been used throughout the ages. It is common folk wisdom that, when one is confronted by a situation that seems impossible, the thing to do is to step away for a while, or "sleep on the problem," in order to return with a fresh perspective. This is a simple method of achieving reorientation to the problem situation.

Reorientation is a broad and pervasive strategy found in all forms of therapeutic problem solving. In one of his earliest descriptions of the basic strategy of psychotherapy, Erickson wrote, "You present new ideas and new understandings and you relate them in some undisputable way to the remote future" (Erickson, 1941/ 2001b, p. 6). Techniques of reorientation are used to produce a significant change of perspective, which provides new ways of conceptualizing existing situational factors, previous life experiences, or future expectancies. Whenever a practitioner impacts the patient's thinking, or provides a new idea, some sort of reorientation must take place. However, there are some techniques that are successful primarily because of a significant, and sometimes jolting, change in perspective. These techniques serve the strategic purpose of reorienting patients to their life experience and hope for the future.

Viktor Frankl's logotherapy is an excellent example of a therapy that incorporates reorientation as the primary therapeutic strategy. Frankl frequently emphasized the importance of discovering meaning in the face of suffering. To illustrate this point, Frankl described a case in which a single question was used to achieve therapeutic results. The patient introduced himself as a doctor and said that he had suffered from severe depression since the death of his wife, two years previous. He had loved her above all else. Frankl's question was, "What would have happened, Doctor, if you had died first, and your wife would have had to survive you?" The elderly man responded immediately that this would have caused her tremendous suffering. Then Frankl replied, "You see, you have saved your wife from that terrible suffering. You have spared her this suffering, at the price that you now have to survive and mourn her." The man said no word but shook Frankl's hand and calmly left the office. He was reoriented to the inescapable reality of her death. Now he could view it as a meaningful sacrifice for his beloved wife (Frankl, 1996).

Although this is not the strategy for which Erickson is most celebrated, the majority of his case reports contain brilliant examples of reorientation accomplished by means of a single well-timed statement. What happens when a woman examines her body in a mirror with the intention of finding something she has never before noticed? Remember, she is used to finding features that she loathes. Now she must find something different. Just as importantly, how can she deny that there is a pretty figure buried under the fat without first losing some weight to see? She is reoriented from knowing that she hates her body to wondering what is actually there. Figuratively speaking, you can say that her wheels are still spinning because she has not been asked to change her mind about the flab. She has not been asked to put less energy into hating that part of her, that fragment of the body. This case illustrates an important aspect of reorientation. It is a strategy that enables the patient to suddenly discover novelty in the most familiar of circumstances.

While explaining the importance of reorientation Erickson remarked, "Often in psychotherapy a change of reference is all that is needed" (Erickson, 1979). Reorientation is a process of taking the same situational variables and placing them within a new psychological context. The psychological shift often illuminates a new path of escape from a situation of despair. This produces greater resiliency in those who feel overwhelmed by life's problems, which is why most people come to therapy and why *hope* constitutes a large part of the cure.

After over two decades of research on stress there is now a great deal of empirical data suggesting that stress is not caused by events themselves but instead by the way in which those events are interpreted. As explained by Mischel (1984), the mental representations of daily events are shown in research to be more relevant to behavior than the actual events. This fact should seem obvious. For example, a husband coming home late from work might have his behavior understood in a way that provokes sympathy (he works so hard for his family), disgust (he prefers his job over his family), or rage (he is having an affair!). The event does not predict behavior as well as knowledge of how it will be interpreted. The implication of this finding for psychosomatic medicine and psychotherapy is enormous.

Using reorientation, the practitioner is able to provide new ways of viewing the situation and reduce the amount of subjective distress. People who feel imprisoned by a bad situation do not use the energy of the mind and body for healing. Progress is most likely to occur when there is an apparent option to pain or suffering. According to Erickson,

> You want patients to realize that illness is only one part of their total life experience. No matter what the illness, patients can always find something to appreciate about themselves. People are entitled to look upon their illness, or pain, or distress, as part of the meaningfulness of life. They ought not to feel that it is something to be frightened of. Why should any patient be frightened by any

Reorientation

type of illness or disability? They have so much else to enjoy. In therapy, your approach should be to help them understand that they brought into your office a lot more than cancer, or arthritis, or any other type of problem. In talking to patients you should convey to them an awareness of all of the other gifts they have.

(Erickson, 1967)

If the function of healing is to discover previously unrecognized capabilities, then it follows that a change in perspective is an indispensable therapeutic strategy.

Insight

Case report: The woman who smoked four packs a day

A woman came to Erickson for help with smoking. However, her expectations for success were extremely low. She explained, "Your friends have all tried to hypnotize me and they have failed miserably. They have all told me that if anyone could hypnotize me you could. So I have come down to let you fail too." To this Erickson responded, "Well, let's get that over right away. We might as well get my failure out of the way. Because I think you need some therapy for your emphysema."

Erickson had diagnosed the emphysema while listening to her breath. He had heard her labored and strained voice and noticed the way she supported herself with the arms of the chair while leaning forward for air. He soon learned she smoked four packs of cigarettes a day. She kept two cartons in a big handbag, two in the glove compartment of her car, two in the back set of her car, two cartons of cigarettes in her bathroom, two cartons in her kitchen, two cartons in her dining room, two cartons in the living room, two cartons in the TV room, and two cartons in the bedroom. Erickson understood that this was a lady who was not going to run out of cigarettes!

The woman did not realize that Erickson's earlier statement had made her therapy contingent on his failing to hypnotize her. According to Erickson, he did a miserable job of hypnotizing her but worked at it long enough to convince her in the absoluteness of his failure. Then he continued, "Now that we know that I cannot hypnotize you and that question is answered, let's take up this question of your smoking. Let's discuss your reason for doing it." The discussion lasted for two hours but without resolution.

The next day, Erickson told her, "I would like you to do as you did yesterday. Keep your eyes open, your ears open and your mouth shut. I have got a few more things I would like to say to you about emphysema and smoking four packs of cigarettes a day. You are going to see me for only one week [she had flown in from out of state]. And I think that four packs of cigarettes inhaled by somebody with emphysema, such as you have, is folly of an extreme sort. You have got a Master's degree. You are a writer who has published extensively. And it just does not make sense to me."

When it became apparent that she was not willing to protect her health Erickson changed his approach and asked, "Why are you trying to kill yourself with cigarettes?" This question evoked a troubling childhood memory, "Because I killed my father."

She went on to explain that, while she was still a little girl, her father had suffered a massive stroke. He was being cared for in his home and she had sat faithfully at the bedside doing everything she knew to do. Her wishful thinking was that as long as she did not stop looking at her father she would not lose him. Eventually, her attention was distracted and, when she turned back to look at him, he was dead. After hearing her story, Erickson responded with great kindness but with great emphasis, "And shouldn't a little girl be allowed to have a little girl's understanding of a situation?"

In a week's time she was down to four cigarettes a day. Erickson reports that she went back home for Thanksgiving but then came back in December and stayed in town for another week. After the second visit she was down to four puffs a day.

(Erickson, 1963)

The technique of insight-oriented therapy has traditionally been associated with psychoanalysis. When used within that context, insight evolves from a process of critical self-examination in relation to the transference relationship. As explained by Arlow (1989), psychoanalysis enables the patient to overcome inner conflicts through insight. Therapeutic results are produced when the insights are used to constructively alter life situations. In other words, the success of the technique is dependent first upon a critical self-examination, then on a reorientation both intellectually and behaviorally to current life conditions.

Rather than the self-critical approach of psychoanalysis, Erickson's use of insight revolved around the central theme of self-appreciation. In the case mentioned above, Erickson helped the woman gain insight into her emotional response to her father's death. The decision she had made about herself as a child was preventing her from developing a healthy identity. After this reorientation she no longer had to view herself as a murderer or failure to her father, but instead, a scared and loving child.

In almost all of his clinical cases, Erickson would strive to communicate the goodness and resourcefulness of the mind, the understandable innocence of childhood, and/or the miraculous construction of the body. These three postulates all serve the purpose of reorienting patients toward their capacity for resiliency. When patients feel good about themselves, they are more likely to make progress toward any number of useful objectives.

Pat Love, PhD, a nonanalytic contemporary who also uses this technique, has noted that insight does not produce change unless it is accompanied by an intense emotional experience (Love, 2003). Love's explanation for this is biological and focuses on the chemical processes necessary for creating new neural pathways in the brain. From the perspective of reorientation, it seems only logical that a meaningful insight is both unfamiliar and somewhat unsettling. When insight is followed by a bland acceptance of what has been revealed, then it seems unlikely that anything new has been added to the person's view of life.

Erickson's most innovative use of this technique was to develop insight in relation to the *cure* rather than the *problem*. While doing this he would create within the patient a heightened state of anticipation about the inevitability of some type of therapeutic result.

For instance, he might capture the patient's attention by stating his doubts about which day of the week the desired behavior will first occur. These comments were seemingly casual but actually designed to generate curiosity. In order to gain insight into the specifics of exactly how the cure would occur, the patient had to make a recovery. This is the exact opposite of how insight has been commonly used.

One of the most frequent criticisms of psychoanalysis is that insight into the development of the problem only provides further justification for the existing complex: "Ah, no wonder I am so messed up!" Traditionally, insight-oriented therapies have focused primarily on the nature of the problem. Erickson, however, preferred to create *an opportunity for the person to gain insight into the nature of his or her capacity to enjoy life.*

Betty Alice Erickson remembers coming home from school one day and seeing one of Erickson's patients sitting outside on the front lawn. When asked what he was doing, he said, "Dr Erickson told me to sit in the front yard and look at the lawn until I can see all the different shades that create green grass." Betty Alice and the young man then sat together studying different blades of grass and how one side of the plant was different in hue than the other. The time passed quickly and pleasantly. When asked about his patient's assignment, Erickson did not answer.

Many years later, within the context of professional consultation about disturbed adolescents, Betty Alice Erickson again asked him about the young man and his assignment. Erickson asked her to guess. Betty Alice recognized that the man was a drug addict. Her guess was that this was a way for him to begin to notice pleasure in everyday life—an insight that he didn't have to use drugs in order to get a high. The exercise helped the young man discover that there was infinite variety and enjoyment in life, but those pleasures and joys have to be noticed in order to be realized. Erickson acknowledged her insight with a smile and said, "Stop and smell the roses."

There are many ways of facilitating insight. As described in Chapter 9 (on progression), Erickson would sometimes orient the person to a point in the future when the problem would be resolved. He would then ask them how this recovery was achieved, thereby producing insight in the form of pseudo-hindsight. When used this way, it is not the accuracy of the prediction that is most important but rather the power of the idea that some type of change is possible.

As seen in the example at the beginning of the section, Erickson used the concept of the unconscious behavior as a means of finding explanations for otherwise unexplainable behaviors. His question, "Why are you trying to kill yourself with cigarettes?" was both alarming and a cue to find new explanations for the patient's current behavior. She realized that she could not keep doing what she was doing and that she had no further need for the behavior. When Erickson commented, "And shouldn't a little girl be allowed to have a little girl's understanding of a situation?" another important reorientation was achieved. Because of her fragile condition it was important to make certain she would not punish herself for believing such an absurd idea. Erickson's comment also carried the implied suggestion that she could now develop an adult's understanding of the situation. In her case, the insight was instantaneous.

On occasion, Erickson found that his patient might spend as long as three months waiting for the insight to develop. During this time the patients might be building up courage, reorganizing thinking in related matters, or waiting for some external event to provide the necessary stimulus, such as a holiday or the anniversary on which something significant occurred. As said by Erickson, there is always a purpose served by time (Erickson, 1952). After all, the power of insight is not in recovering memories from the past but in deciding on a new direction for the future.

Reframing

Case report: Overwhelmed by beauty

> One of Erickson's medical students came to him with an urgent problem. He had married a very beautiful girl and was unable to produce an erection for consummation of the marriage. For two weeks he attempted sex unsuccessfully. In contrast, he had been

very active sexually prior to marriage. After two weeks of a miserable honeymoon, they came back and his wife consulted a lawyer about an annulment. He came to Erickson distraught. Erickson asked to see his new bride and suggested that he solicit the help of some mutual friends who could intercede and help gain her cooperation with the visit. According to Erickson, "She was feeling horribly bitter."

Upon arrival at Erickson's office, her husband was told to wait in the hall. After listening to the woman tell the story from her perspective, Erickson asked her, "Have you thought about the compliment your husband has given you?" She wanted to know what he meant.

After emphasizing the fact that she had been nude at the time of his impotence, Erickson stated, "Well, evidently he thought your body was so beautiful that he was overwhelmed by it, completely overwhelmed. And you misunderstood that and felt he was incompetent. He was incompetent because he realized how little capacity he had to appreciate the beauty of your body. You go into the next office and think that over." The husband was called in, allowed to tell his sad story, and then Erickson told him the same thing. Erickson reports that the young couple nearly stopped the car on the way back to Detroit in order to have intercourse. This was the only intervention that was needed.

(Haley, 1985, Vol. II, pp. 118–19)

"It is not the things themselves which trouble us, but the opinions that we have about these things."
– Epictetus, first century CE

Reframing is a technique that provides an opportunity for the reinterpretation of existing events or situations. Watzlawick and his colleagues were among the first to define reframing as altering patients' perceptions of the problem, its solutions, or their resources in such a way as to reinforce therapeutic interventions. "What turns out to be changed as a result of reframing is the meaning attributed to the situation, and therefore its consequences, but not its concrete facts" (Watzlawick, Weakland, and Fisch, 1974, p. 95).

Reframing is similar to insight in that it also produces an "aha" moment. When it is used effectively there is a sudden reorientation followed by a rush of emotion. The essential difference is that in the case of insight there is a forgotten event that has yet to be processed from an adult perspective or perhaps an event in the future that has yet to occur. In the case of reframing there is usually some type of negative interpretation that has become paired with a specific situation, thereby creating avoidance or resistance. Reframing the situation allows new associations to be established as old problematic thoughts are linked to new reference points. As a result, the reinterpretation provides options for responding that were previously unavailable.

This process could be described as a form of cognitive reconditioning. Stimuli that were associated with negative cognition are broken off and paired with a new more pleasant thought or idea, resulting in a reorientation to the situation. Another way of saying the same thing is that the circumstances remain the same while the meaning of the event is altered.

Reframing is a valuable clinical technique that has been described as a central principle of cognitive therapy (Clark, 1986). Perhaps the most common and widely used reframing technique is one of normalization. Patients most often come to the practitioner seeking someone with expert knowledge, so a judgment about the seriousness of the problem is expected. Although the patient may not come straight out and say, "Is there any hope for me?" a hesitation to reveal much about oneself suggests the possibility of this type of fear. Normalization occurs when the practitioner responds with a statement such as, "Yes, I am familiar with this issue. One of my most successful patients initially complained about the same thing you have described." This statement accomplishes two things simultaneously. First, it provides hope that *something* can be done and, second, it reframes the initial complaint as behavior associated with "successful" responses to therapy.

Normalization is a process of taking a stimulus that has been alarming (and has thus generated negative responses) and assigning a new positive meaning to that stimulus. This was illustrated by Erickson in a case with an adolescent girl who had been brought to him with hysterical chest pains. Prior to this she had been X-rayed, had her chest examined, had been palpitated, and treated with medication. After she had lain in bed for three months, feeling fearful about her future, Erickson used one session to ask her some questions about the sensations in her chest. Then he explained to her that as a doctor he knew it was normal to feel different while developing breasts. After being reoriented to these sensations in her chest, the girl progressed with what was essentially normal development and experienced no further difficulties (Erickson, 1962a). Of course, the use of normalization should be restricted to difficulties that are problematic primarily because of the alarm that has been associated with them, instances where the person has overreacted. It would be a serious error to attempt to normalize a problem that is not fully understood or one that is possibly linked to organic pathology, such as unusual headaches, unexplained pain, or abrupt changes in mood/personality that occur without situational explanation.

In addition to normalizing a problematic experience, reframing can also be a means of transforming shame into pride. This was demonstrated masterfully by Erickson during consultation for the US Army. It was during the time of World War II and, although bedwetting did not prevent men from being accepted into the army, it did create some logistical problems. In order to protect these men from the wrath of their fellow soldiers during basic training, they were all assigned to a special barracks. The sergeant of this barracks consulted Erickson because he desperately wanted to be relieved from this assignment. There was no pride to be found in being an army bedwetter, or in being the sergeant of 600 bedwetters. However, his orders were that, as long as the men continued to wet their beds, he would continue to be their training sergeant. He had already tried every form of punishment for this bedwetting that he could think of, and nothing worked.

Erickson explained that, by the time a man with this habit reached the age of eighteen, he had been punished by his parents, his family, his friends, and society for wetting the bed in more painful ways than either Erickson or the sergeant could imagine. Therefore, the bedwetting had to be accepted and ignored. It had to become just an incidental factor in a whole situation that was unpleasant. The only way for the young soldiers to escape the

unpleasant situation would be to eliminate the incidental symptom that was keeping them in that situation.

Erickson reframed the situation for the sergeant, and subsequently
for the soldiers, when he suggested that the bedwetting barracks
could no longer be identified as just the bedwetting barracks. It
had to be transformed into the hardest damn barracks on the
whole training base. Having the men get up at 4 a.m., to run 25
miles with a full pack as punishment for bedwetting would not
work. Instead, the task was to be performed with the sergeant
insisting, "I train my men in this barracks in this way!" That meant
that the sergeant had to participate in each and every difficult and
painful exercise he gave the men.

The sergeant agreed. The orientation was shifted so that bed-wet-
ting was no longer the issue. Training was—and the training in
that barracks exceeded the most difficult training in the military. A
25-mile run, in full military gear, became routine. The sergeant
joined them as they ran, and did vigorous calisthenics, and then
scoured the barracks, all of this before breakfast. Next there were
several hours of the most difficult training the base had to offer.

Soon, the sergeant's barracks became known across the base as the
hardest-working, toughest training barracks in the army. Many of
the men would do anything to be transferred to a barracks where
they weren't required to put in a full day's work before 7 a.m. and
stopped wetting the bed so they could be transferred. Those who
remained, however, could, for the first time in their lives, stop living life as "bedwetters" and start viewing themselves as capable
men. Those who remained in the barracks had reason to feel a special sense of pride, as did the sergeant. As Erickson later commented, "This really separated the men from the bed-wetters"
(Erickson, 1958e). Although there was some change in the situational variables, much of the drilling done by the men was already
being performed, prior to Erickson's consultation, under the label
of punishment. The primary intervention was a shift in meaning:
the sergeant was now in command of the *toughest* barracks in the
army.

Short remembers a useful reframe as a five-year-old child.
Following an emergency operation, the doctors explained to his

parents that they could not be certain their boy would regain the ability to walk. During a painful rehabilitation process, Short's mother reassured him, "The doctors had to put the tubes in your leg because there was a very bad blood clot. It is a miracle that you can still use your leg. God sent angels to protect you. He must be saving you for something really special!" This open-ended suggestion was reinforced when, at the age of eight, Short fractured his skull. Following the visit to the doctor his mother explained, "The doctor is amazed that you are still alive! God still has his angels protecting you. He must be saving you for something really special in life." Rather than feeling vulnerable or damaged after these potentially traumatic events, Short felt empowered. The reframe that came naturally from a mother's love and faith contributed greatly to her son's resiliency. Future threats to his survival only became further evidence that his life was endowed with meaning and purpose.

This same sort of reframe can be seen in Erickson's work with Rebecca in Chapter 3 (see p. 15). The experience with the attack dog and its owners was an overwhelming situation that left her feeling vulnerable and inadequate. Erickson was able to reframe the situation so that she could feel pride in the goodness of her body.

Reframing is a good means of creating a positive future orientation. It is especially useful in cases where it is almost certain that the patient will experience some form of relapse. After all, most learning occurs in a zigzag fashion rather than a straight line of progression. An important objective is to enable the patient to progress past the point of relapse without giving up. Most therapy will ultimately fail if the patient does not have the resiliency to tolerate normal human shortcomings. Once the patient is oriented correctly toward the possibility of relapse, then this behavior can be beneficial. In fact, Erickson enabled his patients not only to accept the possibility of relapse but to eagerly anticipate it as something that would bring the patient one step closer to success. Erickson often used the analogy of a car rocking back and forth while trying to get out of the snow. The idea of moving backward in order to get a fresh head start was used to communicate the idea that failure can be a necessary component of improvement. In this way moments of weakness are suddenly transformed into evidence of progress, enabling patients to maintain greater resiliency and hope, even during their weakest moments.

The acknowledgment of the patient's original perspective is a vital step in reframing, which the novice practitioner might not fully appreciate. Although it sounds like a reasonable thing to do, accepting something that you hope to alter sometimes feels counterintuitive. A prime example was described at the beginning of this chapter. If the therapist wants to persuade a patient to feel less hatred toward her body, why start by acknowledging how much she hates her "fat" body and all of the "blubber" that is on her? If a woman said she hated her big fat thighs, how could any caring therapist then discuss her body in terms of "big fat thighs?" The reason is that, if the practitioner starts off by rejecting the goodness and validity of the patient's view, then the patient is likely to follow this example and reject the practitioner's views or, even worse, accept the therapist's rejection of the patient's own ability to perceive reality. All sorts of complications, including a meta-neurosis (a complex about one's complexes), can follow such a rejection. When patients feel truly understood, they can stop explaining themselves to others and start considering new ways of viewing the world.

In the case of the newlyweds, sex had most likely become associated with thoughts of inadequacy and failure, for both the bride and groom. Instead of becoming excited by the possibility of sex, there was an increasing sense of dread felt by the groom and resentment from the bride. Erickson's reframing of the situation suddenly broke off the feelings of failure and created the opportunity for the groom to physiologically acknowledge his wife's beauty. After all, if he merely told her she looked beautiful, she would have no way of knowing he truly meant it. He had been very active sexually prior to marriage. Because of this history, she might have suspected that he had used the same line with women before her. However, the involuntary nature of his suffering was beyond question. Following this therapeutic reorientation, she was able to feel more potent than any other female he had ever encountered. At the same time, he had the opportunity to keep his inadequate erection and she could feel beautifully sympathetic toward him. Of course these new associations are more likely to produce the type of reciprocal excitement that is highly conducive to sex. Thus, a win–win scenario was created, regardless of whether the groom achieved his erection.

It should also be noted that the apparent simplicity of Erickson's reframe is a little deceiving. Clever as Erickson's reinterpretation was, it might not have been successful had he not first established himself as someone who fully understood this young couple's needs and desires. It is evident in Erickson's work that *he placed a high priority on assessment* and was *careful to study thoroughly and understand patients' perspectives and their subjective views of reality.* As he made clear in his lectures, Erickson did not communicate new ideas or create new associations until the patient's reality was fully acknowledged and appreciated. After all, if the reinterpretation does not feel like an exact fit to the patient, the idea will be rejected and the technique rendered useless.

Externalization

Case report: Big Louise

While working at the psychiatric hospital in Rhode Island, during the time of prohibition, Erickson learned about a violent patient known as Big Louise. Big Louise was six feet six inches tall and had worked at a speakeasy as a bouncer. Her favorite hobby was walking through the city of Providence in search of a police officer who was alone. She would then beat him up, often breaking an arm or even both, thereby sending him to the hospital. Eventually, the chief of police took Louise to court and had her declared insane and dangerous to others.

Big Louise did not like being in a mental hospital. Her complaint was, "I do not want to be locked up with a bunch of loonies!" Once a month she would go on a rampage, resulting in a great deal of destruction. Before she met Erickson, the only treatment given to her was to send in a contingent of twenty male attendants to overpower her. Some of them suffered broken arms, which added to the problem. After she was overpowered the nurse would give her an injection of a strong tranquilizer, known for the nausea it created. Erickson described the drug's effects and the intense feeling of retching, stating, "For about twelve hours you are tying very hard to vomit up every thing you ate all last year." After receiving the drug, Big Louise would be locked in a seclusion room with nothing but a mattress, which she always tore up, adding to the amount of damage.

After hearing these details, Erickson went to introduce himself to Big Louise. He told her that he would like a nice favor from her. He asked that before going on the next violent rampage she sit on a bench and talk with him for fifteen minutes. She responded suspiciously, "While I am talking to you the male attendants will rush in and overpower me." Erickson responded earnestly, "If you will just sit and talk with me, I personally will see to it that nobody, absolutely nobody, interferes with you." She reluctantly agreed.

One day, Erickson got the call, "Big Louise wants to talk to you." When he entered the ward, she was pacing up and down in front of the bench. Erickson sat down and she sat beside him. "Are you going to have the orderlies gather up and rush in and hold me down?" Erickson said, "No, Louise. I am just going to talk to you. After 15 minutes, you can do anything that you please. And I will see to it, personally, that nobody interferes with you."

Erickson was still new to New England, so he started talking to Louise about springtime there. Louise kept watching the ward door. After about ten minutes, Erickson gave a discreet signal to the nurse, who then placed a phone call.

Suddenly over a dozen female student nurses rushed onto the ward. All of them were giggling as though they were out for a good time. One of them grabbed a chair and smashed all the windows out on the West side of the ward. Another one grabbed a chair and smashed out all of the windows on the East side of the ward. Four nurses rushed to a table and broke off all four legs. Another one rushed to the telephone and yanked it off the wall and broke the receiver. The nurses had been instructed by Erickson to do as much damage as Louise had done in the past.

While they were having a wonderful time, Big Louise began pleading, "Girls, girls please don't! Don't do that! You mustn't do that!" She could not stand to see others behaving the way she had behaved. After the nurses were finished and the ward thoroughly demolished, Big Louise turned to Erickson and said, "Please, Dr Erickson, don't ever do this to me again." Erickson responded, "I promise I will not do it again unless you make it necessary."

Two months later, as Erickson was making his rounds, Big Louise came to him and asked, "Dr Erickson will you get me a job in the hospital laundry?" Erickson said, "You want a job in the laundry. You smashed things up pretty bad when you first came in. I will get you a job in the laundry provided you behave yourself." Louise was desperate. "I will do anything to get off this ward full of crazy women." Erickson sent Louise to the hospital laundry and she did very good work. Two months later, she was discharged as a patient and hired as an employee.

(Erickson, 1980b)

Externalization is a class of techniques that achieve reorientation by allowing the patient to gain an external view of his or her problem behavior. The very behaviors that are most strongly endued with emotion are somehow disconnected from the self so that the individual can better evaluate those actions. Most people have had the experience of feeling justified in their own behavior until the same actions are seen in someone else and, from that external perspective, the behavior appears entirely unreasonable. Most parents have had the unpleasant experience of watching their own bad behaviors imitated by a child. As with all other methods of reorientation, externalization is stimulus for thought that, as a consequence, can produce an entirely new emotional reality.

Erickson skillfully provided his patients with a new, external view of themselves. For example, while working at a psychiatric institution Erickson arranged an introduction between two delusional patients, each of whom believed he was the one and only Jesus Christ. Erickson sat them on the same bench so that each could tell him how crazy the other sounded. After several days of dialogue, one of the patients said to Erickson, "You know, I've been thinking it over. He claims to be Jesus Christ, and I know he is crazy, and you know he is crazy; that's why he keeps saying he is Jesus Christ." Eventually the man was able to give up his delusional thinking, leave the hospital, and on occasion would visit the other Jesus to see how he was doing (Haley, 1985, Vol. I, pp. 229–30). In other words, each patient began looking at himself from a position outside of his own seductive belief system, and did not like what he saw. One of the important benefits of externalization is that it provides patients with an opportunity to reconsider their own identity and perhaps experiment with a new one.

The most dramatic examples of Erickson's using externalization involve the development of hypnotic dissociation. This approach allows the patient to experience some aspect of him- or herself as if it were a separate reality. Obviously, to experience oneself a part from one's own body is a major reorientation.

One of Erickson's most celebrated cases involved a single encounter with a man who was deeply discouraged by life. Erickson identifies him as Harvey.

Case report: Harvey

Erickson describes Harvey as feeling miserable about the way others treated him yet unable to do anything to correct the situation. He was underpaid for his labor, workers blew cigarette ashes across his desk and blocked his car in the parking garage, and there were other small abuses. Harvey responded with miserable helplessness. His only means of escape was to become ill and stay home from work (see the explanation of learned helplessness, which we encountered in Chapter 11, p. 154). Although Erickson's intervention was much more complex and multifaceted than what is described here, hypnotic dissociation was a key component in the progress that was achieved.

The intervention took place in a seminar hall with an audience of doctors. Using hypnosis, Erickson suggested that Harvey could hallucinate several crystal balls. He then asked Harvey to look into one crystal ball and to see a little boy, viewed from the rear. Erickson said, "That little boy must be pretty unhappy … I wonder why. He looks as if he's very, very unhappy. You look at him and tell me where he is." Harvey responded, "Why, that's a little kid about six years old, and he's sitting in his desk at school. The teacher just walked away. She's got a ruler in her hand. She must have been punishing him."

Erickson then shifted Harvey's attention. "All right. Now look in that crystal ball up there. I think you'll see that same little boy. What's he doing?" Again Harvey saw a boy who was exceedingly unhappy. After a series of questions, Harvey looked into the crystal and said, "Why, it's that six-year-old boy coming home from school. He's still got some unhappy feelings. I wish I could see his face, but I suppose it isn't important. He's still rubbing his face— at least, looking at him from behind, that's what he seems to be doing. There are some policemen there, and one of them is holding a revolver. The boy rushes in to see what it's all about, and the policeman has just shot his dog." Erickson then shifted his attention back to the first memory, "But the boy was crying in school, before he found the dog killed. Why was he crying in school?" Harvey responded, "I don't really know, but I've got the most awful feeling in my left hand. And I know just how that boy feels. It feels as if somebody took a ruler and rapped me on the hand for writing with my left hand."

While Harvey was still in a trance, Erickson gave him permission to write using whichever hand he chose: "I'm going to give you a piece of paper and a pencil, and I want you to write your name the way that six-year-old boy would have liked to write."

While Harvey was distracted with his writing, Erickson instructed the doctors in the audience to be complimentary of the writing. These comments were ignored by Harvey. After again securing Harvey's attention, Erickson gave him the following posthypnotic suggestion: "Anybody who tells you that you have written anything is nothing but a damned liar—and you tell them so. Make no bones about it. Just tell them they are damned liars." Erickson awakened Harvey and asked about the writing. Harvey insisted that he had not produced it. Erickson then turned to the audience and asked who wrote it. When the doctors stated that Harvey had, he told-off all of the doctors in the audience, just as he had been instructed.

This pseudo-conflict eliminated any performance anxiety Harvey might have about his writing and enabled him to have the added experience of "telling off" a room full of authority figures. Because his aggressive behavior was the result of a posthypnotic suggestion, it was not Harvey but Erickson who had responsibility for behavior, thereby affording another level of dissociation. After all, it was the hypnosis that "made" him do it.

Once Harvey demonstrated that he could stand up for himself, an antidote to helplessness, the behavior became a permanent part of his repertoire. It was as though a cork had exploded from a bottle. The next day Harvey went to work and demanded better treatment from his fellow workers. He demanded and received a raise from his boss. Harvey went to his psychiatrist and said, "You know, I'm 32 years old and I think it's about time I got a girl. Don't you think so?" The psychiatrist responded, "Well, you know, I've got nothing to say about that. You'll have to consult Dr Erickson." And Harvey said, "To hell with Dr Erickson! I'm going to get a girl." At the time Erickson reported this case, Harvey was happily married and still feeling good about his new empowered identity.

(Erickson, 1977/2001)

How many other ways can externalization be achieved? The list seems practically endless. All that is required is some avenue for self-observation, which circumvents the normal associational cues linking the behavior to the existing identity—in other words, an opportunity to see yourself, at a time when you cannot be yourself. For example, a person who is used to ignoring criticism about his hostile behavior suddenly becomes concerned after accidentally overhearing an honest conversation about the unpleasant nature of his impact on others. He stands outside of himself at that moment because no one is talking to him. As he listens to a description of his actions outside of the emotional context in which they spontaneously occurred, he is given an opportunity to consider what is necessary and appropriate. This is a piece of informal therapy that occurs naturally on a daily basis.

This technique acts as such a strong catalyst for change that it has been incorporated as the backbone of many modern therapies. For example, narrative therapy teaches its practitioners to "externalize" problem behaviors by encouraging patients to objectify, and at times personify, issues that they experience as oppressive (White, 1988). In other words, the patient might be asked to describe the problem behavior as if it were its own entity, separate from the identity of the patient. The patient might be asked to give the problem a name, use imagery to describe its appearance, describe its demeanor, and perhaps even describe its motives.

This technique is not new. Long before narrative therapy, practitioners of Gestalt therapy were creating dialogues between the patient and the externalized problem-self. Once the undesirable portion of one's self is externalized it can be examined, and eventually rebuffed.

Impact therapy also relies primarily on reorientation and externalization. However, rather than using imagery, impact therapy achieves the reorientation by using physical props as a placeholder for personal realities. In a case reported by Beaulieu (2002) a piece of trash was skillfully used to help a severely traumatized child. The boy had become electively mute after witnessing the horrific death of his brother. Beaulieu used a bag of chicken, which had become rotten while traveling in her car, as a prop to help externalize his feelings. She let him know that, awful though the contents of the bag might be, she was strong enough to see and smell what was inside the bag, because it was her job. Tapping into the natural curiosity of a child, Beaulieu and the boy untied the knot together. She commented that the contents of the bag had been well contained but now needed to come out. The little boy got tears in his eyes, began to cry, and then eventually began talking. While untying the knot, the boy was aligned with Beaulieu in action, and therefore by implication was strong enough to handle the horrific mess.

Sculpting, as described by Virginia Satir, and psychodrama, as described by Jacob Moreno, are additional methods for taking any thought, hope, wish, or behavior and putting it outside of one's own person. In fact, a microcosmic version of externalization is achieved any time a practitioner engages in reflective listening, using exact quotations from the patient (Rogers, 1961). If the patient's behavior is also being tracked, and stated back as a mini-narrative of events, then it becomes almost impossible for him not to become reoriented to his statements and behaviors. This combination of tracking and reflection has been shown to produce immediate beneficial effects. This method of intervention is taught to Boy's Town staff as the most helpful method of responding to disturbed adolescents who have become angry or violent (Connolly, et al., 1995).

A similar effect is achieved in therapy when the behavior in question is recorded on tape and then played back at a time when the emotional wave that produced the action has subsided. This is not an exhaustive list of the modern therapies that incorporate this technique but it does provide a picture of its relevance to the clinical endeavor.

And exactly what is the experience that occurs when a person goes to see really good theater? For the story to have an impact there must be at least one character on stage with whom the audience can identify. That figure then struggles with life issues that somehow reflect one's own battles. The drama becomes compelling when you as a member of the audience see yourself from a different perspective. Indeed, this is essentially what Erickson accomplished when he had Big Louise sit beside him and watch the hospital staff destroy the day room. The event was timed to occur at the moment when she was ready to perform these same actions. Thus there was no escaping the fact that, in this drama, each member of the cast represented her. And in seeing her behavior from this outside perspective, it suddenly became intolerable. From that day forward there was no possible way that Louise would feel the same about her violent outbursts.

Reorientation in time

Case report: The woman who had her dolly smashed

> While still a student attending predoctoral lectures at the Menninger Clinic, Erickson was asked to conduct hypnosis with the wife of one of the doctors, who had been acutely depressed for six months. No one was certain how to treat her. The argument was going back and forth, "Should she be analyzed … should she be given supportive therapy?" Up until this point she had been handled through sedation. Young Erickson was approached by the doctor, who said, "I am going to resign at the end of next month because I cannot teach someone how to handle my wife." The doctor was desperate: "I have got to do something about her. She is

becoming more depressed and more suicidal. I have to provide her with a nurse throughout the entire day. So why don't you put her in a trance and see what you can do?" Erickson agreed and said he would conduct the treatment in front of the entire staff.

The woman was in her mid-twenties and intelligent. Erickson began talking with her about her problem. She insisted that she did not like her depression. She did not like her suicidal ideations. She was motivated to get well but simply did not know how. Erickson detected a tremendous amount of emotional ambivalence and, in response to his probing and with tears streaming down her face, she developed a trance state. Having disoriented her to time and space, Erickson told her, "There are several hatreds, disappointments, and unsettling emotions that you can tell to a total stranger, even in public. So let's say you describe a few of them to me. I am a total stranger."

After this she looked upon Erickson as if he were a crowd of people. She was completely unaware of the audience. She did not know if it was summer or winter. This allowed her to talk about quite a number of hatreds, disappointments, and frustrations. She talked about her brother smashing her favorite doll: "He killed my dolly!" She had a great deal of resentment toward her older brother. She also described her rivalry with her older sister over who got the best grades at school.

After she expressed that set of resentments, Erickson said, "Now there are a lot of personal things, private things. You do not have to verbalize them sitting here with me, a stranger. You can let the verbalizations move through your mind at a silent level. So let's sit here for half an hour while you really think through all the things you would not say to the general public. These are things you would really like to say to someone who would be willing to be your therapist."

The next day, she told the nurse who had been assigned to her, "You don't really need to stay around. I am not the least bit suicidal." Erickson conducted this treatment in 1930. Fifteen years later, at the end of World War II, the woman contacted him again by mail. She explained that she was very pleased with the way she stood up to all of her fears and anxieties while her husband was in active service overseas. She was caring for several children at the time. In describing her recovery she stated, "I am very, very pleased."

(Erickson, 1965a)

As with most of the strategies described in this book, it is not necessary to look beyond the domain of common sense to understand the importance of temporal relations as a technique for achieving reorientation. Almost everyone is familiar with the consoling comment, "Years from now we'll probably look back on this and laugh." This statement is repeated generation after generation because it is generally true. Time puts a new perspective on the events of the past, events yet to occur in the distant future, and immediate situations that can pass slowly or with great speed. These phenomena are known respectively as age regression, forward progression, and time distortion. Each is a technique of reorientation in time that promotes new intellectual and emotional understanding.

Although Erickson's use of hypnotic regression and progression often seemed magical, as if a time machine had been created, the technique is more correctly understood as a form of *highly motivated speculation*. And what is the best way to speculate on an event from the past, or the future? The most effective way is to close one's eyes and become fully absorbed in the reminiscence. Lovers have been doing it for centuries. They become "lost in thought" as they muse over the first kiss or dream of a wedding day.

Ordinary schoolteachers can be masters of time distortion. Most of us can remember at least one teacher who was capable of turning fifteen minutes into five hours! After a while of being in that class your head might have felt compelled to drop down to your desk. As you began to lose contact with the immediate surroundings, you might have experienced regression or progression as your thoughts drifted backward or forward in time. You remember the fun you had during the weekend, or eagerly anticipate the upcoming summer vacation. Suddenly, your moment of highly motivated speculation is interrupted as you are reprimanded for daydreaming in class. Sound familiar? *Perhaps the simple act of reading these sentences momentarily took you back in time.* Seeing that reorientation in time is nothing new, and certainly not a magical technique. The ordinary practitioner can do a better job of allowing this natural process to take place. The most crucial skill comes in the selection of a topic that is of vital interest to the patient.

The clinical application of regression and progression was developed by Erickson as a means of achieving a subjective reorientation to a topic of concern. Topics that are of great interest to the patient include questions such as, "What is the most appropriate treatment for your problem?" Using a method he called the *rehearsal technique*, Erickson was able to accomplish an internal reorganization of behavior while simultaneously gaining a clearer understanding of the patient's needs. While describing this process of mental rehearsal, Erickson explains (1958g, p. 107):

> Subjects reoriented from the present to the actual future ... can often, by their "reminiscence," provide the hypnotist with understandings that can readily lead to much sounder work ... it permits elaboration of hypnotic work in fuller accord with the subject's total personality and unconscious needs and capabilities. It often permits the correction of errors and oversights before they can be made, and it furnishes a better understanding of how to develop suitable techniques.

Erickson believed that the ability to affect a person's subjective experience of time was a tremendously important clinical tool. As he explained, "You can reorient the person to the past. You can reorient the person in relationship to the future. You can reorient the person in relationship to his body" (Erickson, 1955a). Erickson described such an instance while working with an amputee who could not adjust to the idea that he had suffered the loss of a leg. Erickson used hypnotic age regression to reorient him to the time when he had both legs. Once the man was absorbed in that recollection, Erickson had him speculate on the question of how he would respond if sometime in the future he had an amputation. This issue was discussed between him and Erickson at length with the focus on how he would adjust if this were to occur. Erickson used the reorientation to raise with him the various questions of adjustment that he knew would develop within the patient and to discuss these problems in a hypothetical manner. This reorientation allowed the patient to consider the topic without too much distress. In the end, it was the patient who developed the solution for how he would deal with the problem of amputation. As explained by Erickson, "From that reorientation you can evoke their capacities for good adjustment and the rejection of their own patterns of maladjustment" (Erickson, 1955a).

Time distortion is a technique that Erickson frequently used in the alleviation of pain. Again, his hypnotic application of the technique seems almost magical, until it is explained within the context of reorientation. While working with cancer patients or those suffering from incurable neurological disorders, most of which could not be alleviated by medication, Erickson would often teach time distortion in the form of time expansion and time contraction. His basic approach was to expand the moments of comfort, so that five minutes passed very slowly, and then contract the moments of pain, so that fifteen actual minutes passed as if it had only been a matter of seconds. In educating his patients this way, he ensured that the person became less focused on pain and more on this issue of time. *More importantly, the orientation to pain was shifted from one of dread and helplessness to one of active correction.*

An important point to understand is the reason it is so important for the patient to believe he can do something about his pain. Consider the following. A small boy is hauled in to the doctor for a shot. Fearful of the needle, he begins to panic and is therefore held down by several adults while receiving the injection. His experience of pain will be tremendous because of the psychological components of fear and helplessness. There is absolutely nothing he can do about the impending pain. Now consider the experience of the same boy while he is climbing a tree. His skin is torn by rough bark as he scrambles up the trunk but the boy does not notice the injury, not until he goes inside the house and sees that he will have to explain to his mother how his trousers became torn. This is an everyday occurrence that reminds us that the pain stimulus is not as significant as the person's psychological orientation to the pain.

Erickson sometimes used a slight change in perspective to initiate both forward progression and time distortion. As Betty Alice Erickson remembers his suggesting, "Instead of looking at what you're doing, look at the ending. How can you make it better?

How can you make it more of what you want? How can you make it more lasting? How can you make it more productive?" This provides a controlled use of dissociation. The immediate task becomes more distant as the future goal is given greater attention. This special focusing of attention on future outcomes also implies the undertaking will end successfully. As most will agree, difficult tasks seem never-ending. But, when one focuses on making the end more of what one wants, a new time-limited orientation is achieved.

More power is added to the technique of forward progression when an experiential exercise is employed. While empowering his patients to imagine and describe their own future, Erickson occasionally would use hypnosis to create hallucinated "crystal balls" so that the person could gaze into the future. Sometimes he would use more than one, "placing" imaginary balls all over his office. This technique was particularly absorbing because it required the hallucination of a crystal ball before fantasizing a vision of the future. Knowing that the exercise could end with a hypnotic amnesia allowed patients to explore thoughts that might have been avoided otherwise.

After studying Erickson's work, Steve de Shazer devised a similar technique, which he calls "the miracle question." The miracle question is essentially this: "If you woke one morning and discovered that a miracle had occurred and your problem was solved, how would your actions change?" According to de Shazer the essence of solution-focused therapy is the miracle question (De Shazer and Berg, 1997).

This question acts as a catalyst for temporal reorientation. In order to describe the miracle, patients project themselves forward in time. The significance of this seemingly simple technique is further underscored by Dolan (2000): "We must be careful because what we don't ask is often more powerful than what we do ask. That is why in therapy it is dangerous when we do not ask patients about their future. This sends the message that they don't have one. And, it is very difficult to defend yourself from a message of which you are not consciously aware."

While summarizing what she considers the essence of solution-focused therapy, Berg explains (De Shazer and Berg, 1997):

> Patients only look at it from one way, the way that gets them stuck. So we give them another way of looking at it. They are in the same situation, but turning it just a small degree helps them look at things from a different angle. And I think that is where the solution comes from.

This explanation represents the essence of the strategy of reorientation and reflects the nature of the therapeutic approach pioneered by Erickson.

As for the doctor's wife with the severe depression, it is at first difficult to see what Erickson did to help her. The use of hypnotic age regression was certainly important to the process. As Erickson explained in a paper, the most direct route for dealing with a problem is to reorient patients to the point in time when their original maladjustments first appeared (Erickson, 1939/2001). He used age regression to help her access emotional states that were very troublesome for her and the situations to which they belonged. Another important aspect of the therapy is that it was performed in front of an audience. Why did Erickson want her to view him as a "stranger" and as a crowd of people? This was an important part of her therapy. She needed to know that she could express herself aloud on difficult subjects in public. To help facilitate this Erickson gave her the idea that she could privately review all of her emotions as if she were talking to a therapist (Erickson, 1965a). Her therapy was both experiential and virtual.

The general application of reorientation

As a father teaching resiliency, Erickson would greet his children when they came home from school and ask which side of the street they had walked on, what manner of walking they used, and whether they had tried different routes. He wanted his children to know that there are many paths to be discovered and that each has its benefits. He discussed the subtle differences in each path, the fact that some are more pleasing than others, and that each has its own sights. When a person has only one way of doing things, then any obstacle to that path can become an overwhelming problem. In contrast, those who explore many paths are better prepared to reorient and approach a problem from a new angle.

As can be seen in the techniques listed in this chapter, there are many different ways of achieving reorientation. Each technique has its own benefits. The skillful clinician will explore many different methods while seeking out those that are emotionally appealing to the patient.

In order to help the patient become more aware of all the different angles from which a problem can be approached, it is often helpful to include an experiential component. Erickson would often incorporate physical movement in this therapy, with patients encouraged to change chairs or to walk in and out of his office, or sent out to walk in the desert or climb a mountain. Physical reorientation often helps facilitate psychological reorientation.

Small simple gestures can also have a strong impact. For example, the therapist might invite the patient to sit for a while in the therapist's chair and imagine momentarily that she is her own therapist. The meditative experience can be enhanced by having the patient close her eyes and wait silently for new thinking to develop. This would be a good technique for someone who admires the power associated with being in the therapist's position. It would not be a good technique for someone who is struggling with boundary issues. Whenever possible, techniques should be individualized to fit the person and the situation. The task of the therapist is to recognize which method will work best with a given individual. This is accomplished through ongoing clinical assessment.

While considering the proper use of this strategy, it is vitally important *not* to undervalue the patient's perspective of the problem and of the path needed for problem resolution. Erickson almost always began therapy by carefully observing and accepting the patient's view of the problem. It was from this point that he and the patient embarked on a journey of change. For Erickson, it did not matter if the patient's ideas were inaccurate or unscientific. For example, there was an illiterate man who wanted dental hypnosis and could easily develop oral anesthesia but, each time the dentist touched his mouth, the anesthesia evaporated. After seeking more information from the patient it became apparent that the "eye teeth" were the source of the problem. Because of the name given to these teeth, the man believed they were connected with his eyes. As long as he could see what was happening he felt that his teeth were not fully anesthetized. Erickson's solution was to simply tell the man to close his eyes (Erickson, 1962a). *In the provision of psychological care, the beginning point must be where the patient feels the need exists.*

Along these same lines, it is important for the therapist to recognize that there are always more ways than one of viewing events and that the opinion of the therapist may not be entirely correct for a given individual. It is the patient who must decide what to make of his or her life circumstances. An example of a well-intentioned but tragic misuse of reorientation was communicated to Dan Short by Ellen Taliafero, MD.[1] A woman came into a physician's office with severe injures to the head. After interviewing her, the physician recognized that she was in a physically abusive relationship. She was not ready to leave the relationship so the physician had his nurse cancel the rest of his appointments for the day. He spent the time convincing the woman that she must leave the relationship and go to a shelter. She finally agreed to the doctor's view of things and was in the process of leaving the house when the abusive partner discovered what she was doing and killed her. Although this is something that might have been bound to happen, the fact that she was acting on the doctor's instructions when the death occurred placed the responsibility for this tragedy on his conscience. Unfortunately, the doctor underestimated the importance of listening to this woman's opinion of what she felt she could safely do. This example emphasizes the point that reorientation is *not* a matter of telling other people what to think or do, which is coercion. In contrast, reorientation is a nondirective strategy for broadening possibilities and providing new options for the *patient* to choose from.

The last point to be made about reorientation is that of pacing. The more fundamental the shift in thinking, the more time people need for reorientation. The concept of reorientation fits well with the

---

[1] Author of *Physician's Guide to Domestic Violence*, Volcano Press, 1995.

Tolmanian notion that all creatures derive much behavior from a cognitive map of the environment. These are the expectations that allow us to operate more efficiently. However, when there is a change in the external world, then healthy adaptation will require a reorganization of the cognitive structures used to represent these external events. This is a neurological process and, as is true for all biological processes, the reorganization and construction of new associations requires time. This is one reason why the skillful clinician waits and allows patients to develop insights at their own pace.

Chapter 12

Utilization

Utilization, the final and most distinctive strategy in this book, is the defining hallmark of Erickson's clinical approach. If Erickson's philosophy of healing were to be condensed to the single statement "help patients recognize the goodness of their mind and body," then utilization is the most direct manifestation of this mandate. The dynamics underlying the strategy are simple though its clinical application can seem counterintuitive. As will be seen in the following case examples, Erickson's ability to make full use of this strategy was both profound and inspiring.

Case report: Jesus

> While Erickson was on staff at Worcester State Hospital, in Massachusetts, there was a young man who insisted he was Jesus. He paraded about as the Messiah with a sheet draped around him. Furthermore, he felt strongly that it was his mission to impose Christianity on people. This behavior resulted in complete alienation. The patient continued his attempts to engage others socially but in an aggressive manner that ensured his rejection. Acting as a sort of father figure, Erickson told him, "Since your purpose on earth is to serve mankind, there is a task you can do that will serve people." The first mission Erickson gave him was to smooth the dirt on the tennis courts, "God surely did not intend for all those lumps to be in the tennis court." After some time, Erickson approached him again: "I understand you have experience as a carpenter." Because Jesus is said to have been a carpenter, the patient had to accept this statement. Erickson then instructed him to serve mankind by using his carpentry skills to build a bookcase for the psychological laboratory. The patient eventually became the laboratory handyman.
>
> (Haley, 1973, p. 28; Gordon and Myers-Anderson, 1981, p. 43)

It is interesting to speculate on the many possible reasons for becoming seduced by the idea of being Jesus. In most cases, delusional thinking represents a failure to cope, a narrowing of perceptual learning and processing. This type of intense inward focus allows the individual to ignore threats posed by an environment that is otherwise beyond control. And just as interesting is the capacity of those who are not psychotic to also shut themselves off from reason. As Erickson explains (Erickson and Zeig, 1977/2001, p. 1),

> When you understand how man really defends his intellectual ideas and how emotional he gets about it, you should realize that the first thing in psychotherapy is not to try to compel him to change his ideation; rather, *you go along with it and change it in a gradual fashion and create situations wherein he himself willingly changes his thinking* [our emphasis].

Or as one of Short's fourteen-year-old patients jokingly stated, "I'll see it *when* I believe it."

Regardless of the clinical concern, most people have a tremendous need to be *known* and *accepted*. The clinical significance of this interpersonal dynamic is reflected in Erickson's approach. As noted by Haley (1973), the liberal use of acceptance was Erickson's fundamental approach to human problems whether or not he was using hypnosis. In order for acceptance to feel genuine, the patient must know that the therapist is fully informed of the hidden parts of self associated with shame or disgust. This knowledge is then followed by positive recognition and a readiness to utilize that aspect of the person. Erickson's philosophy of healing was characterized by *his attention* to the goodness of the patient's mind and body. This paved the way for utilization and a shift in the client's focus of attention. After all, how much hope can there be if the individual's constitutional resources are regarded as flawed or useless?

In moments of weakness, people often require additional amounts of external validation. For many, a lifetime is spent seeking out someone to help them believe in themselves. But providing the level of acceptance they require is not always easy. For example, when dealing with a person who is losing control of his sanity, it is easy to feel that he should listen to the reasoning of others and not his own. One might ask, "What good is accomplished in allowing him to continue to think that he is Jesus?"

As another example, when providing treatment to someone with numerous psychosomatic illnesses, it is tempting to dismiss her right to experience both suffering and care. When hearing statements such as, "You are not really sick: it is all in your head," the patient feels terribly invalidated, which might be the issue that caused her to seek care in the first place.

While you are responding to people who come to *you* for help, it feels natural to focus on what *you* can do for them. Yet when focusing on *your abilities* and *their problems*, an implied message of therapist superiority and patient inferiority is communicated. This is why utilization requires a special type of acceptance that sometimes seems counterintuitive.

In order for therapy to be successful, there needs to be a willful participation of the patient and employment of his or her physical and psychological resources in the task of living. With willful action comes responsibility and with responsibility comes increased control. Therefore, the practitioner accepts the patterns of behavior that most strongly characterize the individual. In many cases, this means accepting the pathological behavior targeted for change. As Erickson explained, it is important to demonstrate to patients that they are completely acceptable and that the therapist can deal effectively with them regardless of their behavior (Erickson, 1959/2001). Thus, the will of the patient is ratified as the practitioner strategically constructs a series of positive outcomes using existing personality resources. The result is a transformation of negative energy, aroused by the problem situation, into a more positive and constructive application of that energy.

The term "utilization" is used to describe this clinical strategy because it points toward the meaningful involvement of the patient in the healing process. Utilization comes from a willingness to recognize and use the patient's behavioral, emotional, and intellectual predispositions as a fundamental treatment component. The analogy Erickson often used to explain the concept was that of a person who wants to change the course of a river. If this person opposes the current by trying to block it, the water will merely go around him or he will be swept away. But, if he accepts the force of the river and diverts it in another direction, the power of the river will cut a new channel (Haley, 1973, p. 24). Some incorrectly refer to utilization as if it were a single technique. As Erickson explained, there are numerous techniques of utilization (Erickson, 1959/2001, p. 1). What these techniques have in common is the therapeutic bind that is created by employing the behavior that dominates the patient (*ibid.*). *Paradoxically, acceptance can be used as a compelling force for change.*

A reoccurring theme in Erickson's teaching was the importance of eliciting the participation of the patient's entire personality (Erickson, 1958b). Accordingly, the clinician must watch for opportunities to make use of robust aspects of the patient's personality, which might include the utilization of personality characteristics that are initially irksome. This clinical task requires conscious effort and above all else, the proper attitude. This attitude was described by Erickson when he explained (Gilligan, 2001, p. 25),

> I don't know how the patients are going to respond. All I know is that they *will* respond. I don't know why. I don't know when. All that I know is that they will respond in a way that suits them as individuals … I can comfortably wait for their response, knowing that when it occurs I can accept and utilize it.

In order to function with this degree of flexibility, the clinician must wholeheartedly embrace the idea that there is more than one way to solve any problem. This includes problems encountered by the patient and/or problems encountered in the office as the therapist attempts to help the patient.

Utilization is as much a point of view as it is a process. If the patient threatens to slap the therapist in the face (see p. 115), then this energy can be accepted as something to be utilized as part of a cooperative endeavor toward the clinical objective. When the therapist knows that he will utilize everything the patient says and does, then it is possible to implement the therapy with great confidence. For example, a child was dragged into Erickson's office and left in the middle of the room screaming at the top of his lungs. Erickson calmly waited for the boy to stop for a fresh breath of air. Then he used the momentary pause to let out his own loud scream. The boy was stunned. Erickson explained, "You took your turn. Then I took my turn. Now it is your turn again." He and the boy took a few more turns screaming and then they decided to take turns talking, instead (Erickson, 1980a).

This illustrates the type of therapeutic environment necessary for utilization to occur: "First, you will show me your behavior and I will accept it, then I will respond with a behavior that you can accept." As Erickson explained, the initial acceptance of the patient's behavior, and a ready cooperation, stimulate the patient to further effort (Erickson, 1959/2001). Once patients are engaged in this way, and as the pattern of give and take continues, they become more and more committed to a relationship aimed at achieving clinical objectives. Because patients' personality traits are welcomed by the therapist, utilization diminishes the likelihood of a power struggle. Rather than being met with confrontation, such as when patients are told they *must* change flawed aspects of themselves, there is an attempt to evoke more of who they are and what they are doing. When patients are invited to act in accord with their own constitution they are less likely to feel coerced into change. Not only does this diminish resistance to therapy, but more importantly it places the locus of change where it belongs: inside the patient.

Any aspect of the individual and his or her life situation can be utilized in therapy. The objective of utilization is broad rather than specific and symptom removal is not the primary aim. The sort of thinking that allows only one acceptable outcome is too linear and does not permit much maneuverability. Thus, utilization is *not* focused on changing the individual but instead there is a striving toward acceptance. *A previously unrecognized potential is employed to achieve any outcome that will be helpful or appealing to the individual.* In other words, the clinician utilizes some aspect of the personality or current situation for some positive purpose. This then provides the spark that ignites the healing process. The recognition that healing occurs from within makes the meta-teleological position imperative, that is, the primary goal of the clinician is to facilitate the activation of patient goals (see p. 29).

For Erickson, utilization was an important means of providing patients with options. He then trusted they would make the choice that was right for them. For example, Erickson had a patient, at age fifty, who had accumulated numerous behaviorally influenced diseases such as Buerger's disease, diabetes, cardiac disease, and high blood pressure. Before coming to Erickson, he had been in psychoanalysis five days a week for eight months. During that period of time his blood pressure went up 35 points, he began smoking four times as many cigarettes as before, and he gained 40 pounds. After hearing this, Erickson told the man to close his eyes and repeat his story from beginning to end. The man thoroughly described his inability to fight a compulsion toward self-destructive behavior. The man was then encouraged to *outline in great detail the therapy that he thought to be indicated*. After having him say the treatment plan four times, Erickson pointed out that he had offered no advice or corrective suggestions, that every aspect of the plan came from the patient himself, *and that he would find himself under the powerful compulsion arising from within him to do everything that he thought was indicated*. A year later, the man returned in good physical shape and asked Erickson to treat a friend in the same way he had helped him (Erickson, 1964/2001a). This deeply respectful approach allowed Erickson to utilize whatever came into his office and thereby offer his patients a strong sense of confidence in *their* ability to respond favorably to treatment.

In summary, the strategy of utilization represents the essential character of Erickson's clinical approach. It is a methodology that puts a unified mind and body in motion to heal itself. *Utilization acts as an antidote to neurosis by fostering greater self-acceptance.* In the same way that muscles must be used to remain healthy, the various aspects of the patient's personal reality should be employed rather than rejected. That personal reality might include resistance to therapy, aggression toward the therapist, or the desire to maintain remnants of the old symptomology. Although not all forms of utilization are paradoxical, it is often the case that by accepting a behavior you begin the process of altering it. When rigid problematic behaviors are incorporated into the process of therapy, it helps ensure the patient's participation. By targeting the problem behavior for utilization, value is brought to formerly rejected aspects of self. Part of Erickson's genius was his ability to recognize such aspects of the patient's personality, behavior, and situational influences and employ them in therapy.

As can be seen in the case of the man who thought he was Jesus, the technique of utilization can be understood as a process of transformation. This can include transforming weakness into strength, or nonvolitional behavior into meaningful activity. It is done with great respect for the patient and provides clinical benefit when the transformed behavior helps the patient develop increased hope for the future.

Utilization is not trickery and is certainly not meant to show off the cleverness of the clinician. It is meant to enhance the subjective sense of self that develops within the patient. When Erickson directed the man to engage in acts of service, he made use of the delusional thinking in such a way that a new self-concept could emerge. Rather than being ridiculed or marginalized for his delusional thinking, the man was put in a position of being appreciated by the doctors at the hospital who enjoyed tennis. Furthermore, the bookcase he built stood in the laboratory as a monument for everyone to see. The handiwork represented something good that had come from inside of him and from the work of his own hands. The man's self-image changed to reflect a greater sense of value. Eventually the power of the delusional thinking faded as real-life rewards became available.

Simple bind

Case report: *The woman who wanted to waste time*

> A woman who weighed 255 pounds came to Erickson with the problem of obesity. Uncomfortable with male authority figures and highly resistant toward anyone attempting to manipulate her, her resistance to change had caused her to abandon a previous therapist. When it became apparent to Erickson that she did not want to talk about issues that were relevant to therapy, he described the situation as he saw it: "I believe that no matter what I do, you will continue to insist on wasting the therapy hour." This idea appealed to her. She worked to convince Erickson that he was correct. Erickson then conceded that she was in fact manipulating

him and that it was a privilege for which she had to pay. According to Erickson, her payment included gradual improvement in her overall condition.

(Erickson, 1959d)

Erickson often emphasized the importance of not trying to control other people. He felt that the more helpful thing was to create a therapeutic opportunity that had strong appeal for the patient. This opportunity was presented as a gift; it was something that *bound* energy to action.

All of the techniques described in this chapter create a motivational bind. The bind described in this section is "simple" because it is intended to be straightforward rather than paradoxical (i.e. "You want X, so do Y"). This is a utilization of situational factors. A simple bind is a technique that employs unrealized desires in order to create sufficient motivation to activate and sustain problem-solving behaviors. New associations are created as the fulfillment of a strong desire is made contingent on the development of necessary problem-solving behavior.

A simple bind is a matter of recognizing what a person would like to do and then linking that to some therapeutic outcome. This is a utilization of personal values and desires. The concept is not so different from the idea of offering a carrot to a pony so that he will move forward. However, for one pony it may be an apple, for another a banana, and radishes for yet another. In other words, rather than a generic reward, the patient's existing desires are employed. A patient who likes to save money is helped to quit smoking by pointing out exactly how much money will be saved each year. Another who always insists on winning is pitted in a competition against someone else who is also trying to quit smoking. And yet a third person who needs to stop smoking and wants to get in better shape is told to climb up a mountain trail each morning and breathe the fresh air. It is this highly individualized approach that makes the technique a matter of utilization rather than mere behavioral conditioning. Not only does the behavior change, but implicit in the approach is an acknowledgment and affirmation of the patient's personal system of meaning and values. *Who the patient is becomes an important part of therapy.*

And why do Erickson's children love canned spinach to this very day? As Betty Alice Erickson explains, while they were still young, Erickson would tell them they were too little to eat spinach. This was a little upsetting for the children. Mrs Erickson would then come to their rescue by arguing that they *were* now probably big enough to eat canned spinach. Erickson's children clearly wanted to be bigger and older. So they responded to this bind by sitting up in the chair as tall as possible, trying to look older and more mature. Eventually, Erickson would give in, expressing his many doubts, and allow the children to have *a bite*. Betty Alice still remembers begging for spinach, cold from the can, and still eats it that way. The bind also created a nice reward for Mrs Erickson as well. Her opinion was the one that prevailed. It structured a situation in which everyone was bound to win.

Decades ago, when abortion was a dangerous and illegal activity in the United States, Erickson needed to persuade a young couple not to follow through with plans for a hasty termination. However, he found that he was entirely unable to persuade them using logic and reason. He eventually acquiesced and ended the meeting with the admonition, "Whatever you do, don't name your unborn child." Erickson knew the couple's relationship had been forbidden by their parents, and as a result had increased their desire for one another. Similarly, Erickson provided another forbidden action. The initial bind was simple: *if you want to have an abortion, do not think about a name for the baby*. But utilization of the couple's refusal to heed Erickson's advice then led to the next more profound bind: *if you have a name for a baby you need to have a baby to give it to*. As the couple began to personify the child by giving it a name, they also began to think about how much love they might have for their unborn baby.

Another example could be described as *taking the wrong side of the argument*. This bind is simply an argument against change that utilizes patients' desires to take up the other half of their own ambivalence. When talking to students who were failing in school, Erickson often would say, "It is your right to decide how much you will learn and I do not want you to learn one thing more than you want to learn!" This provides a strong contrast to what they are accustomed to hearing from their parents: "You better get your grades up or else!" When interviewing inhibited patients Erickson often said, "Do not reveal to me any secrets that you are not comfortable sharing." Rather than thinking about how difficult it is to share information, the patient is left thinking about what he or she would like to share (Erickson and Rossi, 1981). After all, rarely does a patient come to therapy in order to say nothing. This is no more acceptable than a child considering the possibility of having nothing to show for her time spent in school.

As with any type of therapeutic bind, for this approach to work a meaningful contingency must exist. But, unlike the use of a carrot, while taking the *wrong* side of the argument, the patient is initially given something to move away from. Of course, if you move away from one thing, then you are by implication moving toward something else. For example, once while teaching, Betty Alice Erickson had a demonstration subject make an extraordinary request, "Hypnotize me, Betty, and make me quit cheating." He had not been able to commit to a single relationship his entire life. Because of his infidelities, his first wife left with his son and moved to another country. His second wife left before having a child. His third wife left before having a child. His current wife, the fourth, had just given birth to a baby boy. The man knew that if he cheated on her, again, she would leave with their baby.

Betty Alice inquired about his childhood and discovered that he had grown up uncared for, basically living on the streets. Considering this impoverished past, she felt that his current position in life and positive orientation toward people was rather remarkable. After using both formal and informal trances to intersperse numerous suggestions about the significance of his accomplishments, Betty Alice asked in passing, "Who is going to teach your son to be a man?" Before he had time to respond, the question was quickly dismissed, "Well, maybe your son will work as hard as you did and become a good man." This was obviously the wrong side of the argument. The man did not want to lose his son. The thought was so overwhelming that he suddenly burst into tears. The audience was stunned. Two years later, the man contacted Betty Alice to let her know that he was still married and committed to raising his son.

A great paradox in the art of change is that, whenever you attempt to *take* a problem behavior away from the patient, a natural tendency is for the patient to hold onto it more tightly. This territorial behavior is especially apparent in the three-year-old child who clings tightly to any object you attempt to grab. In therapy, this can become a counterproductive bind that clinicians should strive to avoid. Fortunately, this process can be reversed so that a simple bind is created that motivates the patient to engage in problem solving behavior by his or her own choice.

One such method is to advise a patient to *postpone any further improvement*. The clinician's statement might sound something like this: "Your problem is a complicated one and therefore your progress needs to be gradual." The postponement can be argued for the sake of a spouse, other family members, or so that there is proper time for adjustment. The important point is that the clinician does not accidentally communicate the idea that the patient is incapable of progress. Instead, the patient is made to feel ready for action and ready to defy others' expectations by making progress at their own pace. Of course, if you are making progress at your own pace, the implicit bind is that you must make progress. When this is done correctly, the emotional effect of postponement is a substantial increase in desire for continued improvement.

As indicated above, people tend to want what they cannot have. This is one of the most deep-rooted characteristics of human behavior. The best way to make a child want to eat spinach is to move it just beyond reach. In a similar manner, the patient becomes excited about the possibility of recovery but, when the clinician moves it just out of reach, there is an instinctual desire to pursue it with even greater determination. In some instances, the individual feels so compelled to achieve a speedy recovery that recovery acquires a nonvoluntary status. There are several instances in which Erickson had patients come back and apologize to him for their failure to postpone their recovery any longer (Erickson, 1962b).

Double bind

Case report: Johnny's big chassis

As mentioned earlier (see p. 21), twelve-year-old Johnny was dragged into Erickson's office by his irate parents. Erickson confronted the parents for their harsh treatment of the child and quickly dismissed them from his office. It should be noted that this occurred many years ago, prior to child-abuse laws and before protective services were established.

After marveling over Johnny's size, five feet ten inches tall and weighing 170 pounds, Erickson took some pressure off Johnny by stating, "Your parents want you to have a permanently dry bed right away, and that is simply unreasonable. In the first place, you have been too darned busy to bother to learn to have a dry bed. You have a great big beautiful frame, with great big powerful muscles to handle it. Your chassis is one that took a lot of energy to build and it is almost as big as your father's and you are only twelve years old. It took an awful lot of energy to build a body as big and strong as the one you've got, and you didn't have any energy left over for such unimportant things as a dry bed or mowing grass or being a teacher's pet. But you will soon be full-grown, bigger than your father, and you haven't got far to go to beat him. Then you'll have all that energy and horsepower you have been putting into growing to spread around to the other things you want, like a permanently dry bed. In fact, you are so close to being finished with building that great big powerful body that you've probably already got extra energy to spare."

Having gotten his attention Erickson stated, "As for your bed wetting, you have had that habit for a long, long time. And this is Monday. Do you think you can stop wetting the bed and have a permanent dry bed by tomorrow night? I don't think so and you don't think so. In fact, nobody with any brains at all will think that sort of thing. Do you think you will have a permanent dry bed by Wednesday? I don't. You don't. Nobody does. In fact, I don't expect you to have a dry bed at all this week. Why should you? You have had a lifelong habit. And I just simply don't expect you to have a dry bed this week. I expect it to be wet every night this week. You also expect that and we are in agreement. I also expect it to be wet next Monday, too. But there is one thing that really puzzles me. And I am really absolutely and thoroughly puzzled. Will you have a dry bed on accident [*sic*] by Wednesday or will it be on a Thursday? And will you have to wait until Friday morning to find out?" Johnny listened attentively to these ideas. The look on his face indicated that these were thoughts he had not considered before. Then Erickson gave Johnny an important assignment, "You come in and tell me next Friday afternoon whether it was Wednesday or Thursday, because I don't know. You don't know. The back of your mind doesn't know. The front of your mind doesn't know. Nobody knows. We will have to wait until Friday afternoon"—which was Johnny's next scheduled appointment.

Friday afternoon, Johnny came in beaming. He told Erickson something that Erickson described as delightful: "Doctor, you were mistaken. It wasn't Wednesday or Thursday. It was Wednesday and Thursday!" Erickson responded cautiously, "Well, just two dry beds in succession does not mean that you are going to have a permanent dry bed by next week. Why, half the month of January is gone! Certainly, in the last half of January you can't learn to have a permanent dry bed and February is a very short month."

After giving Johnny some time to absorb these ideas, Erickson continued, "Johnny there is one thing I would like to have you understand. I don't know if your permanent dry bed will begin on March 17th, which is St Patrick's Day, or if it will begin on April Fool's Day. I don't know. And you don't know either. But there is one thing I do want you to know. When it begins it is none of my business! Not ever, ever, ever is it to be any of my business."

In follow-up, Erickson reported that Johnny was fully grown and practicing medicine. He had gotten married and had a boy of his own. He was kind to his son. At the time of follow-up, he was six foot four inches and weighed over 240 pounds, all of it muscle. He was big enough to look down on the little old man who used to rub his face in the wet bed. Erickson reports that he looked down with tolerance and amusement. According to Johnny, "Dad did the best he could. He didn't know any better."

(Erickson, 1952/2001a, 1962b)

How is a double bind different from a single bind? As implied by its name, it is more binding. There is less room for escape. The technique can be described as a sort of *benevolent* ambush. Its use is based on anticipation of predicted future behaviors, which are employed as a therapeutic contingency. This is a matter of utilizing foreseeable outcomes. In some instances, Erickson would even employ the patient's resistance to therapy as part of the double bind (Erickson, 1952/2001a). When asked to explain his use of the double bind, Erickson provided the following formula: "You present therapeutic ideas to people and make them contingent on the things that are going to occur" (Erickson, 1962b). Using the double bind, the clinician can introduce new problem solving behavior by making it contingent on the expression of highly probable thoughts, feelings, or actions. This type of contingency is normally not recognized by the patient. It is a complex form of commitment in which the person is bound not only by their words and desire but also by firmly established patterns of behavior.

An elegant example of a therapeutic double bind can be seen in the following interaction between Erickson and a young boy. "I know your father and mother have been asking you, Jimmy, to quit biting your nails. They don't seem to know that you're just a six-year-old boy. And they don't seem to know that you will naturally quit biting your nails just before you're seven years old. And they really don't know that! So when they tell you to stop biting your nails, *just ignore them*!" (Erickson, Rossi, and Rossi, 1976, p. 66). The first contingency in the bind is easy to recognize. The boy will turn seven. His birthday was just a few months away, and that was something that was bound to occur. The second contingency, which was a utilization of existing behavior, is more difficult to see. If the boy had really been listening to his parents when they told him to stop biting his nails, he would have stopped. Therefore, when Erickson made the therapeutic outcome also contingent on Jimmy's continuing to ignore his parents, he used, in a positive way, a behavior that was highly likely to occur. As explained by Erickson, this double bind created the opportunity for Jimmy to give up nail biting on his own. Accordingly, Jimmy later bragged about the fact that he quit a whole month before he turned seven (Erickson, Rossi, and Rossi, 1976, p. 66).

The logic of the double bind is simple and straightforward. Yet its application requires some practice. Having read the previous section, you should know how to use a simple bind in order to get a child to eat spinach. But how would you foster good eating habits using a double bind? "Try not to think too much about the spinach until after you have eaten enough of the other good food that is already on your plate. Then we can talk about whether or not you will get a bite of spinach." With every bite the child puts to his mouth he becomes more and more invested in eating that spinach. And how much is enough? The more bites the child takes to try to convince the parent that he has eaten enough, the more invested he becomes in finishing what is on his plate. This benevolent ambush creates a psychological situation that is not easy to escape.

The use of double bind in therapy can be as simple as giving recognition to the current state of affairs faced by the patient. Patients initially set themselves up for a double bind by choosing to come to therapy. Once they make it through the door, without evidence of coercion, there is no disputing the fact that they are committed to being in the therapist's office. As long as they are there in the office, they have to do something. *If therapeutic change is made contingent on finishing the therapy hour, then a double bind is created.* This contingency can be established using subtle remarks. For example, one could say to the anxious patient, "It takes a lot of courage to seek out help and make yourself vulnerable in this way. Just taking this first step is two-thirds of the battle. Odds are that, after leaving this first appointment, *you will not feel as nervous as when you entered*." These statements could be mistakenly identified as truisms. They so closely fit the patient's immediate experience that the double bind is difficult to detect (i.e. you are finishing the session, therefore you will improve).

In the case of Johnny, at the beginning of this section, he initially resisted coming into Erickson's office. He complained that he was tired enough to go to sleep and that he would rather go home. Erickson told Johnny that he could defeat the purpose of the interview by going to sleep and not listening to what he had to say. Johnny willingly came into the office, went into a deep hypnotic sleep, and thereby committed himself to the rest of the therapy process (Erickson, 1952/2001a).

Erickson also used the technique of double bind while soliciting information from certain psychiatric patients, those who withheld vital information, such as the true nature of the problem or desired outcome. To create a double bind under these circumstances, the continued withholding of information becomes the contingency on which progress is predicated. The need to resist ensures eventual compliance. For example, Erickson would insist that such a patient withhold information from him for another week or two. This allowed the patient to defy instructions from an authority figure while at the same time communicating the information needed for treatment (Erickson, Rossi, and Rossi, 1976). The important point to recognize in this and all other instances of double bind is that it represents a full acceptance of the patient's immediate needs. It is this fundamental aspect of the therapeutic double bind that makes it a process of utilization.

There are numerous opportunities for the use of double bind in therapy. Any time the patient is asked to demonstrate a symptom, a double bind is created. The patient wants to be understood and might not recognize that, if he can start something, then at some point he must decide to stop it. Every intentional beginning must have an intentional end. Short attempted to explain this logic to a woman who had come in for help with panic attacks. The panic attacks had been occurring every night for the past five years. She stated that she could afford only one visit and that she doubted that psychotherapy could help with what she believed to be a physical disorder. Hypnosis was offered as a means of safely inducing a panic attack of brief duration. She was horrified by the idea. Short did his best to explain why this would be beneficial, but after some time she won the debate and was greatly relieved to hear that any further talk about an intentional panic attack would be put off until *after the hypnotic exercise was completed*. She went into trance quickly and deeply. During this time, the conditions were created that she identified as being most likely to produce a panic attack: her eyes were closed, the lights were off, and she was in a reclined position. But there were no suggestions about having a panic attack. After waking from trance the woman was insistent that she had listened to every word spoken in order to see if Short would try to make her have a panic attack. The end result was that she *proved* she had the will and resiliency necessary to *choose not* to have a panic attack. This was a utilization of her reluctance to comply with *all* of the therapist's requests. That night she did not experience a panic attack, nor any other night. Several months later she made arrangements to come in for more hypnosis to help with other issues. A good therapeutic double bind is much like the *fork in the road* described by Lawrence (Yogi) Berra, former catcher for the New York Yankees: "It doesn't matter which road you take because eventually you are going to end up at the same place."

Although any attempt to influence others can be seen as manipulative, the therapeutic double bind is not a control-oriented technique. It is not something to be imposed on others. When this occurs, the double bind creates an unhealthy situation that eventually leads to some inescapable punishment, "Damned if you do and damned if you don't" (Watzlawick, 1978, p. 105).[1] In contrast, a therapeutic double bind is tailored to fit the patient's personal agenda. The patient who finds himself in a therapeutic double bind does not feel forced to comply with some demand. After all, it is the patient who sets the therapeutic objectives toward which the double bind serves.

If the therapist has the proper attitude, the double bind is seen as an extension of the patient's right to decide. It is the power of the patient's commitment to healing that makes the double bind effective. Otherwise, the therapist's remarks would just be ignored. As stated in the Introduction, healing is *not* something to be forced on an individual. The therapeutic double bind is instead offered as one of multiple paths toward the outcome that the patient desires. When done correctly, it is an opportunity for patients to realize explicitly or implicitly their innate power to change.

Another important factor is the saliency of the contingency that is established. The contingency must be one that is both convincing and reliable. It must appeal to the logic of the patient and it must be cued by a variable that occurs as predicted. Perhaps this is why Erickson often used the symptom complex itself as the contingency for improvement. What could be more reliable than a

---

[1] It was this destructive form of the double bind that inspired the Bateson team to invent the term "double bind," and identify this negative dynamic as a possible cause for schizophrenia (Bateson, 1972). This theory did not have sufficient empirical support and has since been rejected.

problem that will not go away? Rather than dread the moment when the patient's symptoms would inevitably reemerge, Erickson happily awaited the outcome of what is essentially a win–win paradox. The patient can spoil the therapeutic directive by not repeating the symptomatic behavior, in which case therapy is successful. Or the patient can repeat the symptomatic behavior and as a result of cooperation with therapy find that the behavior no longer functions as it once did, in which case an impetus for change is initiated.

Erickson's most straightforward example of this process was a description of how he provided some relief for a patient with abdominal cancer pain. In this case, the pain was experienced as a recurring stabbing pain. Erickson responded to the patient's need for comfort by saying, "With each stab of pain you will notice an increase in the warmth in your legs. With each stab of pain you will notice an increasing feeling of *comfortable* warmth in your legs." The purpose of this statement was to help the patient recognize the possibility of experiencing comfortable warmth in some part of his body. Erickson initiated the process of experiencing comfort in a location where there was no cancer. The fact that this new learning was contingent upon the experience of a reoccurring symptom, located in the stomach, made it more likely that the patient would alter his perception of his abdomen (Erickson, 1962b). The man was bound by both the reliability of the stabbing pain and the plausibility that warmth could be experienced somewhere in his legs.

Much greater complexity is evident in cases in which Erickson employed disagreeable aspects of the personality as a contingency for clinical progress. These are instances in which he was able to pit one problem behavior against another. A good example is Erickson's work with a physician who had insomnia. As the patient explained to Erickson, "For twelve years now I have gone to bed at 11:30 p.m. I get to sleep by about 2:30 am. By 4:00 a.m., I am rolling and tossing. I fight it out and I get madder and madder … Life is getting pretty miserable. My wife will not let me in her bedroom at all because she cannot stand my rolling, and tossing, and my swearing about my lack of sleep … I am pretty much at odds with my entire family."

Erickson questioned the man about his early life. He had worked his way through both college and medical school. The man had a great deal of interest in English literature. In college, he had looked forward to the day when he could read all of Dickens and all of Scott. After discovering how busy he had been and how badly he had wanted to read those books, Erickson said, "Now listen, doctor. You have been in practice for many years. You have been too busy to read these books, yet in college you promised yourself you would read them. As long as you are staying awake every night, night after night, just wasting time, as you have been doing for twelve years, why not really stay awake and profit from it? So set up a lamp on the mantle and put a volume of Dickens there. Go to bed at the regular time. If you are not asleep within half an hour, you get up and stand at the mantle so you can read Dickens all night long. Don't sit down. You will fall asleep if you sit down. Get caught up on reading Dickens. Stand there the rest of the night. You can do it. A waitress stands on her feet all day long. You can stand on your feet all night long. *You will only miss an hour and a half of potential sleep at the most. You can afford that* [Erickson's emphasis]" (Erickson, 1962b).

The doctor was convinced by Erickson's logic. For the first three nights he read at the mantle all night long. The next three nights he slept all night long. This became his standard practice. Eventually, he read all the volumes of Dickens, and all the volumes of Scott, and Shakespeare as well. According to reports from the man and from his wife and children, his adjustments to his family improved tremendously. His medical practice also improved tremendously (Erickson, 1962b).

Although this case has been used to illustrate a strategy that Haley (1984) refers to as ordeal therapy, Erickson (1962b) used this as an example of the double-bind technique. First, there was an acknowledgment of the man's personality pattern, which was oriented toward self-punishment. This was one problem. Not sleeping was another problem. So Erickson established a contingency that enabled the man to punish himself constructively any time he wanted. As Erickson explained, "He keeps two volumes at the fireplace to 'punish' himself whenever the occasion arises" (Erickson, 1962b). The desire to punish himself was made useful and the insomnia was made useful. No matter which direction he turned, he was bound to succeed. This is the same formula described at the beginning of this section: *introduce new problem-solving behavior by making it contingent on the expression of highly probable thoughts, feelings, or actions.* The therapeutic value of this technique is not found in illusions of control, but instead in the acceptance and *utilization* of significant aspects of the patient's personality.

The most interesting feature of cases such as the one above is that future occurrences of the problem behavior are not only tolerable, they are transformed into something that is desirable. A similar dynamic can be seen in the case of the patient who had spent eleven years sitting in a wheelchair because of painful arthritis (see p. 7). Because Erickson anticipated the reappearance of severe arthritis pain in the future, he was able to make continued progress contingent on the certainty of relapse. The man was given a seven-day "vacation" during which he was in bed reading books. The double bind fit the patient's logic and provided a greater appreciation for the set of circumstances he had been dealt. He was bound by both the residual arthritis and the demands of a busy schedule to enjoy his time in bed. It was an event that had a definite beginning and end. This helped shield him from a potentially damaging idea that the therapy could provide only temporary relief and that he would eventually have to return to the condition that existed prior to seeing Erickson.

Because small amounts of failure are a part of any endeavor, the prediction of a small failure becomes a double bind when it is linked to evidence of progress. Another example of this is Erickson's work with Cathy, a case previously described on page 63. She was suffering from intolerable pain which Erickson reduced but did not entirely eliminate. It was the experience of unrelenting *minor* pain that produced the double bind. While explaining his use of double bind Erickson stated, "As long as she had distress at the breast area, she had to have numbness elsewhere in her body. And she could keep on wishing I could be as successful there as I was elsewhere. Thus I had all of Cathy's general experience substantiating the numbness of her body … by letting her keep that minor pain; I inferred the success of the rest." The woman had been told by her doctors that she only had a few months to live. The failure of her health was an inescapable reality, so Erickson utilized "failure" as an opportunity to promote her progress.

A very important point to recognize about the use of double bind is that it is not necessary to "make" the patient carry out a directive. Success can be made contingent on a refusal to comply with a therapeutic ordeal. Betty Alice Erickson remembers asking Dr Erickson to help her overcome a longstanding fear of the dentist. Despite good teeth, she had an irrational fear of the dentist. When her children became old enough to visit the dentist, she decided she did not want to model that fear.

Erickson asked her repeatedly to explain why she wanted to overcome this fear, because it hadn't really bothered her up until then. Erickson pointed out that the children's father was not fearful and they could take after him. He had many reasons why Betty Alice did not need to be concerned with the issue. However, she persisted. She really did not want her children to learn this irrational behavior. Finally, Erickson agreed he would help and that in a single afternoon he would cure her fear of the dentist, forever.

First, Erickson had Betty Alice agree to follow his instructions. The instructions were as follows. Make a big sign that reads, "I faint at the dentist's office." Put the sign on a string so it can be worn around your neck. Erickson offered to make arrangements with the family dentist for her to sit in his office. He would inform the receptionist that, if Betty Alice did faint, the receptionist was to ignore her and to tell any concerned patients that everything was all right and they could ignore the situation.

Erickson assured her that if she fainted she would not be unconscious for long and then could resume her seat with her sign around her neck. "You will be cured of your irrational fear of the dentist in one day!" he said proudly.

Betty Alice was horrified, "I won't do it!" Erickson replied, "All right," and turned to walk away. Betty Alice continued to be horrified. "But you told me you would help me overcome my fear of the dentist to help my children!"

Erickson turned and looked at her. "I have given you a way to help your children and you turned it down." As far as he was concerned, the conversation was over.

Looking back, Betty Alice views this intervention as a wonderful success. First, Erickson made certain that her motives were strong. Next, he promised the attainment of her goal. Then he set up a situation with three options, two of which were unacceptable. She could humiliate herself in public or she could not help her children. The third implicit possibility was to cure herself. This was the option Erickson was certain she would take and therefore her success was made contingent on her *refusal* to follow his directive. Although she had asked for his help, Betty Alice did not want Erickson to fix her. If he had, then the gift to the children would have come from him rather than from their mother.

Years later, she asked him why he had structured that situation as he had. He responded that he had great faith that she would be able to figure out the answer for herself and was relying on that. "Worked, didn't it?" he said with a confident grin.

And what is the double bind that Erickson used with Johnny? On what contingency did Erickson position the therapy? The boy knew he had been a bedwetter all his life and that no amount of punishment would make him stop. Therefore, Erickson had to select an even more powerful therapeutic bind. As Erickson explains (1964a),

> Looking at that boy I knew to expect some growth. I could tell by looking at the shape of his face, the size of his hands, and the density of the tissue over his elbows and ankles. His mother was five foot eleven inches tall with a large skeletal frame. She was a large framed woman. Johnny had all the odds in his favor of reaching a height greater than his parents. So I gave Johnny a different kind of view of his body. I gave him a face saving explanation: "It took an awful lot of energy to build a body that size in twelve short years." I called him a "kid." It was friendly. He knew he was only in the 5th grade. In double binds you present new understandings and new ideas and you relate them in some indisputable way to the remote future. Johnny was going to get older. He would get taller. He would get heavier. He would go on to high school. He would go on to college. I did not mention high school because it needs to be the remote future. He went home thinking about becoming a football player rather than thinking, "Am I going to wet the bed again tonight?"

Johnny could not help but to grow and become bigger. That was the physical contingency. However, Erickson also inserted a clever *psychological* contingency. It is similar to the paradox of forcing yourself not to think of the white elephant with bells on its ears. In order to avoid thinking of it, you have to constantly remind yourself of the image. And so the issue of attaining a permanent dry bed was turned into absolute certainty when Erickson made the comment, "It is none of my business!" As Erickson explains, "That was a posthypnotic suggestion that would go with him for the rest of his life." For the rest of his life, Johnny would have to remember not to tell Erickson about his permanent dry bed and *the only way to do that was by having a permanently dry bed*. In other words, the question in Johnny's mind was not "Will I have a dry bed?" The question was "Which night?" and then "What will I say to Dr Erickson once I have a permanent dry bed?" Johnny's continued progress in therapy rested on the probability that he would search for an answer to these questions. And why was the psychological contingency so important? As explained by Erickson, "Therapy is a participatory thing and you better have your patient participate with you" (Erickson, 1964a). The recognition of this fact then reflects the essence of utilization.

Utilization of a minor problem

One of the values of utilization is that it does not matter where it is applied. A person's strengths can be utilized as can weaknesses. In some instances, it is even helpful to use shortcomings that were not originally part of the clinical presentation. If the adjunctive problem is one that can be easily corrected, then a valuable opening is created. In such cases, Erickson would use the resolution of a minor problem as an initiation for recovery from other more complex clinical problems.

Similar to earlier utilization techniques, a very subtle and implicit bind is created when a patient responds favorably to treatment for a minor problem. For years, salesmen have used the notorious foot-in-the-door technique. Before asking a person to comply with a large request, they first ask the person to comply with a small one: "Can I just show you my product?" Research has shown that people are more likely to agree to a large request after they have agreed to a small one (Freedman and Fraser, 1966; Howard, 1990). The bind is implicit. After the successful performance of the initial request, individuals see themselves as possessing certain traits (Freedman and Fraser, 1966). In the context of therapy, patients who respond favorably to treatment of a minor problem see themselves as capable not only of healing but also bound to the healing process for the sake of consistency. Cialdini (1995) refers to this as the consistency rule. "After committing oneself to a position, one should be more willing to comply with requests for behaviors that are consistent with that position" (p. 264). Cialdini prefaces this rule with a quotation from Leonardo da Vinci: "It is easier to resist at the beginning than at the end" (p. 264).

Utilization of a minor problem allows clinicians to employ the challenges of daily living and utilize the successful resolution of one problem so patients can recognize their capacity for resolving other, more complex, issues. It is then the minor task, and not the major clinical problem, that becomes the focus of effort. For this technique to be most effective, the selection of the minor task should be based on whatever the patient believes needs to be improved (Haley, 1984). One of the most eloquent case descriptions of the technique can be found in an article by Erickson, written on the topic of utilization (Erickson, 1959/2001, pp. 24–5). Erickson had been contacted by the parents of a nine-year-old girl because she was failing in reading, writing, and arithmetic. She was also failing socially and withdrawing. When questioned about her experience at school, she would reply either angrily or tearfully in a defensive fashion, "I just can't do nothing." After some investigation, Erickson learned that she had been capable of good scholastic work in previous years but she was less successful on the playground. In her social dealings she was inept, hesitant, and awkward. However, her parents were concerned only about her academic performance.

Because the girl would not come to his office, Erickson met her each evening in her home. After learning that she did not like certain girls because they were always playing jacks or roller-skating or jumping rope, Erickson enticed her into learning how to play jacks. Within three weeks she was an excellent player.

Her parents were very displeased with Erickson's lack of attention to academic matters. Nevertheless, Erickson used the next three weeks to teach her to be a capable roller skater. Next she learned to jump rope. This only took a week. Erickson then challenged her to a bicycle race, which she won. As Erickson reports, "That was the last therapeutic interview. She promptly proceeded to become the grade school champion in jacks and rope jumping. Her scholastic work improved similarly" (Erickson, 1958e, p. 25). At the end of her school experience she graduated with national honors.

As can been seen in this case, Erickson utilized other areas in which the girl suffered from performance anxiety and created an expectation of accomplishment. The initial successes she experienced with Erickson created a new self-image that generalized to multiple areas of her life. Essential elements that contributed to the girl's commitment to continued progress include (1) her active involvement in the therapy process, (2) the fact that she was asked to do something requiring effort, (3) the fact that her victories were witnessed by others, including her brother, and (4) the fact that she felt internally motivated to perform the tasks that Erickson asked of her. These are the same four dynamics described by social psychologists as being instrumental in securing a pattern of consistent responses (Cialdini, 1995). When used therapeutically, these dynamics create a special kind of hope, the type that is likely to result in continued progress. It is the pervasive influence of this technique that makes it so useful.

Symptom prescription

Case report: The boy who eeked

William was a seven-year-old boy who had a reoccurring vocal tic. Once a minute, all day long, he made a noise that sounded like, "eek, eek." His mother, father, and teachers were disturbed by this unyielding behavior. Everyone wanted to know why he made these sounds. Erickson was asked for his assistance, so during a home visit he sent William to his room with medical orders that he should make his eek sound twice a minute rather than just once a minute. This had to be done before he would be allowed to leave his room. Although he initially resisted, William eventually decided to "eek" twice a minute. After a full day of practicing the sound twice a minute, he was told that he ought to watch the clock because, if he did not "eek" twice a minute, he would be sent back to his room. The next day he was asked to try eeking three times a minute. After that, four times a minute. This routine was justified by Erickson's need to study and examine the behavior. Erickson reassured William that it was important to understand why he made the "eek." The boy felt that Erickson was very stupid to need so much time studying his behavior. Within a week, William had taken control of the habit and did not care to have it again. Several years later, his parents confirmed that he not only stopped eeking but also remained free of any other symptomology.

(Erickson, 1960b; Erickson, Hershman, and Sector, 1961, p. 326)

"Sometimes the best way to convince someone
he is wrong is to let him have his way."
—Red O'Donnell, c. 1900–84

The word "prescription" is a term that is commonly associated with the idea of being directed by a doctor to *physically do* something during a *daily routine* for the sake of recovery. It is a ritual of modern medicine in which a bitter pill must be swallowed, although sometimes the medicine may be sweet. This ritual can facilitate healing even without the presence of medicine, as shown following decades of research on placebo therapy. Accordingly, in psychotherapy there are behavioral directives that engage patients in the healing process by making them active participants in the therapy. The therapy that begins in the office must eventually find some application in day-to-day living. For this reason, Erickson would frequently prescribe tasks to be performed outside of the office. This is one way that learnings achieved in therapy are generalized to other settings. It is also a means of securing a commitment to change and expectation of progress.

When the behavioral directive involves the repeated performance of an unwelcome behavior, such as with symptom prescription, the process of commitment is all the more profound. There is no reason to ask patients to do something outside of their behavioral repertoire, which they might dismiss as impossible, when instead they can be asked to do something that they can hardly restrain themselves from. The implicit message behind such a directive is that patients *can and should be who they are*, and, by *doing more* of what they cannot stop themselves from doing, they will make progress toward healing. Under these circumstances, therapeutic change occurs as a byproduct of the patients' experiential learning and out of cooperation with the therapeutic agenda. This is a special subclass of double bind that warrants consideration as a unique and highly developed technique of utilization.

In the broad clinical literature, the term "symptom prescription" is used along with other terms such as "paradox," "paradoxical intention," and "paradoxical directive." These concepts are roughly equivalent. However there are some finer distinctions between differing types of paradox that will be introduced in this section. Of these, "symptom prescription" is the clinical term that most precisely describes the general procedure and fits with its many variations.

Although Erickson was not the only clinician to successfully employ paradox, he was one of the most creative in finding different ways of prescribing a symptom. Some methods described in the existing Ericksonian literature include symptom scheduling, symptom embellishment, symptom displacement, and symptom substitution. All of these have in common a paradoxical directive to continue experiencing the symptom in some way so that change can occur. Two of these can be seen in the case at the beginning of the section. While prescribing the symptom, Erickson *embellished* it by having it occur with greater frequency. He then *scheduled* the symptom by emphasizing the importance of watching the clock and making certain the eeks occurred according to schedule. He then embellished it further by increasing the scheduled number of eeks. Other options for embellishment include increases in the intensity of the symptom, the duration of the symptom, and the complexity of the symptom pattern. As in the case of the boy with a vocal tic, symptom embellishment and symptom scheduling were often used by Erickson as a means of turning the symptom into an ordeal and thereby hastening its extinction (Haley, 1984).

The third variation, *symptom displacement*, involves the reification of external objects. The classic example is when Erickson had a woman leave her airplane phobia in a chair. The symptom displacement was so real for her that she would not allow anyone else to sit in that chair (Erickson and Rossi, 1979). The concept of symptom displacement initially seems somewhat extraordinary. But if one accepts the idea that people do indeed use a defense mechanism known as *projection*, then the technique can be seen as a utilization of this natural tendency. Projection is a spontaneous means of escaping unacceptable thoughts, feelings, or behaviors by attributing them to others. When the projection is intentionally aimed at a benign object, rather than a person, then the symptom has been prescribed and displaced in such a way that progress can be achieved without any social complications.

The final variation of this technique, *symptom substitution*, involves a directive to change the location or topography of the symptom experience. Patients are instructed to experience the symptom in a different part of the body or with different physical features. This technique was more commonly used in cases in which Erickson believed that the patient needed to retain some remnants of the symptom complex. For instance, a schoolteacher who was compelled to have a loaded gun with her at all times was told by Erickson that she *must* have something in her purse that symbolized death and for that reason she was to carry a "loaded" cap gun, no matter where she went (Erickson, 1977b). This is a change in the topography of the symptom, which at the time would not have caused any alarm for parents or other teachers.[2]

In another interesting case, in which Erickson acted only as the consultant, a clinician was able to help a soldier who had a psychogenic paralysis of the arm. Using hypnosis, the soldier was instructed to experience all of the paralysis within his little finger. This way the paralysis did not interfere with his ability to use his rifle (Erickson, 1977a). It could be argued that the paralysis was "displaced" rather than "substituted for;" however, the change in location involved the substitution of one type of paralysis for

---

[2] One should realize this intervention took place at a time when there was no gun violence in the schools and no terror in the airports. With the way society has changed, this specific directive is no longer advisable.

another. In either case, the end result is paradoxical in nature. The soldier began to make progress only after he was told that he must retain some remnant of his problem.

Although the essence of symptom prescription is merely the patient's willful acceptance of a previously unacceptable behavior, thought, or feeling, greater power is added to the technique when using one of the variations of symptom prescription listed above. This provides an opportunity to make slight alterations in the patient's habitual patterns of response. By adding something onto the pattern of symptomatic behavior, such as with symptom embellishment, a subtle process of change is initiated. As the symptom is gradually modified, in some inconspicuous way, the strategy of progression combines with the therapeutic utilization of the problem behavior. This strategic compound reminds us of Erickson's remark that if you can budge a patient one inch this can initiate a process of ongoing growth. In the case of therapy, it is the person's distress that is progressively diminished.

Erickson first started experimenting with paradox in 1930 (Erickson and Zeig, 1977/2001). This was about the time that Viktor Frankl, the founder of logotherapy, was independently developing his conceptualization of paradoxical intention (Frankl, 1939). Similar to Erickson, Frankl argued that paradox provides patients with an opportunity for choice, where before none seemed available. According to Frankl, "… man is by no means merely a product of heredity and environment. There is a third element: decision. Man ultimately decides for himself! And, in the end, education must be education toward the ability to decide" (Frankl, 1973, p. xix). Through the combined use of humor and symptom embellishment, Frankl enabled the patient to self-detach, "to put himself at a distance from his own neurosis" (Frankl, 1984, p. 127). In contrast to Frankl, Erickson's paradoxical utilization of symptoms was highly individualized. Erickson's justification for the technique was linked to the patient's personal goals and objectives rather than an existential doctrine.

One such goal that some individuals bring to therapy is their unstated intention to defy the efforts of a powerful authority figure. For some, the experience of having defied someone as powerful as a well-known doctor is an empowering and perhaps transformative event. If the clinician works from a doctrine of change that does not recognize this as a legitimate goal, both patient and therapist are likely to become caught up in a covert power struggle that produces very little payoff. Under these conditions, it is what the patient *does not* do that is more important.

For example, within the context of family therapy, a girl with anorexia might be told that her illness serves an important "stabilizing" function for the family and that she must continue to refuse food. Previously she was rebelling against the parents' attempt to force her to eat. Now the expectation is that she will rebel against the therapist's directive that she must continue to deny herself food. The hope is that she will return to the next session well fed (Selvini, 1988, p. 218). This is a secondary utilization of the symptom. A more complete or primary utilization would be the use of the patient's need to resist. Although the technique of secondary utilization can help defiant patients bring involuntary behaviors under control, it does not address the needs of patients who are seeking to comply with and gain approval from an authority figure.

In contrast to a secondary utilization of the symptom, during primary utilization it is what the patient *does do* with the symptom that is more important. Using symptom prescription, the therapist accepts symptomatic behavior and then incorporates it in some useful outcome (Zeig, 1992). As Loriedo (1997) explains, "... paradox means to be accepting when patients expect you to refuse. You surprise them. You find a good part of the symptom so you can be confirming rather than rejecting" (p. 19). When prescribing a symptom, Erickson would often find a way to *transform* the behavioral pattern into a means to a desired end. In doing this, he went to painstaking measures to fully and accurately understand the goals and desires of his patients. This enabled him to move his patients closer to the thing they subjectively needed but could not achieve, and he accomplished this using their own methods. As is true of most effective therapeutic techniques, there is a reorientation that takes place as the symptomatic behavior is reframed as something of potential use (Lankton and Lankton, 1983, p. 68).

This primary utilization of the symptom is illustrated in a fascinating case in which Erickson prescribed the symptom of intentionally urinating in bed as an ordeal for a married couple who each had a history of life-long enuresis. It is important to note that these two individuals were very religious, very submissive to authority, and felt a great deal of shame and embarrassment over their behavior. The embarrassment was so much that they had not told each other about the bedwetting. Neither was aware that the other also was enuretic. As described by Erickson, "Their wedding night had been marked, after consummation of the marriage, by a feeling of horrible dread and then resigned desperation, followed by sleep. The next morning each was silently and profoundly grateful to the other for the unbelievable forbearance shown in making no comment about the wet bed." Erickson utilized this spirit of self-sacrifice and their need for penitence, the mechanism that would eventually provide relief from their unbearable shame, by prescribing the ordeal of religiously kneeling in bed together and urinating on their clean sheets, for a period of five weeks (Erickson, 1954/2001). It should be noted that this directive required a lot of time and careful preparation before the couple were actually told what to do. Erickson told them to take a week to think about this choice and that if they followed the directive exactly as he stated there would be no charge for the therapy.[3]

In contrast to a secondary utilization of the symptom for the sake of dealing with resistance, it was important in this case for the couple to do what was asked. After suffering through this ordeal together, there was no question about the distinctiveness of this shared experience or of their readiness to simultaneously stop the behavior. After all, it could have been very humiliating for one to successfully stop the behavior while the other continued. The symptom prescription reaffirmed their unity and uniqueness as a couple, long after the problem had been resolved.

Although most all patients benefit from some form of therapeutic utilization, not all patients are good candidates for symptom prescription. A person who is suddenly cast into difficult life circumstances, such as a wife who is about to lose her spouse to a terminal illness, requires a more supportive type of technique. Similarly, patients who are seeking the outside opinion of an expert do not need to be told to experience more of their problems.

---

[3] For a more detailed description of the case see Erickson, 1954/2001.

Individuals who present with dangerous or threatening behavior are not good candidates for symptom prescription. As Loriedo (1997) points out, it is dangerous and stupid to use a paradoxical prescription with someone who is suicidal. It is almost never a good idea to tell someone to go ahead and kill himself. Skillful practitioners have successfully inserted prohibitive injunctions for those considering suicide but this is not to be confused with symptom prescription. For example, Betty Alice Erickson told one such patient that he must spend his entire life savings before committing suicide. She knew that he was overly tightfisted with his money and that he would be horrified by the suggestion. He refused the directive with great indignation and twelve years later is still doing well and has even more money in savings. He was directed to do something drastic but not something that would result in death.

When there is a character disorder, such as commonly seen in cases that involve abusive relationships, alcoholism, or borderline personalities, symptom prescription should be used with extraordinary caution. Those with a character disorder often require a different type of therapy (Cummings and Cummings, 2000, p. 91). While treating character disorders, rather than reducing internal conflict the clinical objective might include an intensification of internal monitoring and self-consciousness (Short, 2001). For this reason, and for issues of safety, symptom prescription is usually not appropriate.

Symptom prescription has proved to be a useful means of dealing with subjectively experienced problems that patients do not expect to be capable of reducing or eliminating. Those who come to therapy with *specific* complaints about seemingly *involuntary* behaviors are most likely suffering from intense internal conflicts, implicit versus explicit desires that have deprived them of the sense of choice. Ambivalence is one form of internal conflict in which paradox can be used to provide an opportunity to experience choice (Beavers, 1985). Reviewing the research, Frankl (1977) notes that paradoxical intention is effective for those with obsessive-compulsive or phobic conditions. He explains that such individuals tend to be caught up in a vicious cycle of fear and avoidance that only reinforces the problem behavior. Once the behavior is accepted, the cycle is broken (p. 117). Along these same lines, O'Hanlon (1987) has purposed that if the frequency of the symptoms increases as the patient tries to avoid or get rid of them, then some form of symptom prescription is probably appropriate. Similarly, when patients' goals become more and more distant as they strive to attain them, then this is another good indication for symptom prescription (Lankton and Lankton, 1983, p. 69).

In order for symptom prescription to be effective, it is essential to fully understand the underlying dynamics of the problem situation. In some cases, what at first seems like a solution is actually just another variation of the problem. The following case is a highly complex form of symptom prescription in which the core problem is difficult to recognize.

Case report: Perceived impotence

A man came to Erickson overly concerned that he was impotent. Erickson did not believe that this was the true problem and warned the man that there would come a time when he would get an erection and it would happen at a time that was inconvenient for his wife, *at a time when he could not do anything about it.* After leaving the session, and having his erection at an inconvenient time, he returned and admitted to Erickson that he was not impotent. Erickson's next question was, "What is this very, very difficult problem that you had to conceal under the mistaken idea that you were impotent?" The rest of therapy was spent directing the man's attention to abstract issues that were not likely to impact his functioning at home or work.

(Erickson, 1959d)

The problem faced by the man was his neurotic preoccupation with the idea that he might have a disorder. Initially, the point of reference for his thinking was his penis. What developed from this was the fearful expectation that at some crucial moment his penis would fail him and prove to be an embarrassment. Erickson broadened this expectation by creating an opportunity for his performance anxiety to emerge at any time and in any context. Thus, the symptom was not only prescribed but also embellished.

In order to resolve the issue of impotence, Erickson's patient needed to recognize that an unexpected behavior could occur, in his pants. The erection at an inconvenient time enabled the man to want the very thing he once dreaded, a limp penis. There was also a need to understand that he did not have to view his sexual behavior as "the problem." The patient's need to view himself as having a serious problem was also utilized by reframing the limp penis as being just a minor problem. As we know from the preceding section, after successfully resolving the minor problem, the man was now psychologically committed to resolving the next therapeutic issue. With one cure already under his belt, Erickson then enabled the patient to choose the next clinical issue to be resolved. What then followed was a harmless indulgence in neuroticism. Having resolved a minor problem, as well as a much "deeper" problem, greater resiliency was established.

General application of utilization

In contrast to physicians, it has been said that the most important tool of a therapist is his own mind and body. But that is not the position of this book, nor was it a theme in any of Erickson's lectures. Conversely, Erickson argued that it is the patient who is the most important tool of therapy and that it is the patient's lifetime of learning and experience that provides the substance needed to promote progress. Now with the benefit of forty years of controlled outcome research, the importance of recognizing the patient's central role in the change process has been demonstrated very convincingly (Hubble et al., 1999).

It is the central role of the patient that makes the strategy of utilization so fundamental to Erickson's therapeutic approach. When the therapist has this attitude, the patient's imperfections become an avenue toward progress rather than something to fight against. Furthermore, the patient begins to recognize that the therapist not only accepts who he is but also wants to use his existing abilities as a basis for progress. This promotes an inwardly oriented form of hope that is not easily dismissed.

Questions of clinical judgment that are dictated by the logic of utilization include: "Which behavior do I attempt to utilize?", "How can I use behavior that seems destructive?", and "What outcomes should I attempt to achieve with the utilization of a given behavior?" The answers to these questions come from an eye for opportunity. The process of utilization builds as therapy becomes increasingly characterized by acceptance.

As with all of the clinical strategies described in this volume, utilization can be misapplied. The strategy is not likely to be effective if the therapist is not respectful of the patient's right to reject a behavior absolutely. While it is true that patients should learn to be flexible, it is not wise to argue with patients about the usefulness of some behavior they have formally rejected. If a woman never again wishes to walk down the streets of a big city, then there is no reason to argue about this. Rather than send the woman into town for systematic desensitization, the therapist should instead utilize her position by suggesting a walk in the country. Here it is important to recognize the significant difference between a patient who comes to therapy because she wishes to be able to walk in the city again and the patient who informs the therapist that she never again wants to walk in such a setting. *Utilization holds no promise when it is pitted against the will or future good of the patient.*

It is also important to recognize that a therapist should not utilize behaviors that have proved to be highly destructive. After a lecture on this topic, an attendee at the workshop asked Short the following clinical question, "I have a patient who talked his wife into sleeping with him and another man. Now he is paranoid that she wants to leave him for this other man and will not stop obsessing over this possibility. How do I utilize this?" With utilization, there is always more than one correct answer—the act of engaging in sex with multiple partners is not a good focal point for the behavior that will be utilized. Instead, therapeutic utilization features behaviors that involve assets.

With utilization, there is always more than one correct answer. In this case, Short's suggestion was to start by reframing the paranoia into a more constructive orientation: "He cannot stop thinking about his desire to *save* the marriage. Once you get him to acknowledge this, then focus the conversation on what concrete actions he can take toward healing the marriage, and keep him thinking about it. Even if he fails to save the marriage, he has a lot of valuable things to learn during this worthy effort." Rather than attempt to fight against the pattern of obsessing, the therapist can bind it to more productive behaviors. Upon meeting the patient, Short might have changed his mind and utilized a different behavior that represented a richer opportunity. Utilization requires great flexibility and a willingness to revise one's thinking on a minute-by-minute basis.

The logic of utilization applies to any effort to introduce hope into situations that initially seem hopeless. This strategy works only as long as the patient is capable of doing what he is expected to do. Although Erickson used a provocative style of therapy, it is important to recognize that he did not ask the patient to do anything that he was not absolutely confident the patient could do. For example, during hypnotic induction Erickson might ask the person to experience catalepsy (a hand left floating in the air), knowing that any person who holds his head upright throughout the day is capable of balanced muscle tonicity, which is accomplished without conscious intention. In a similar manner, while prescribing therapeutic objectives, he constructed the task using proven behaviors. Rather than suggest the necessity of a behavior that may not exist within the patient's repertoire, he would employ existing *behaviors and beliefs* in a way that allowed the patient to initiate change (Erickson and Zeig, 1977/2001). This is an important caveat that is essential to the process of utilization.

Chapter 13

Conclusion

About the book

During the last several decades, many different theories have been developed in an effort to explain and replicate the pioneering work of Milton H. Erickson, MD. The most useful theories are parsimonious. They achieve a comprehension that is as complete as possible using a minimum of theoretical constructs. The result is a general understanding that will act as a guide for navigating what would otherwise be experienced as bewildering. For the sake of clarity, it is important to avoid the creation of excess jargon and overanalysis of minutiae. In a field that demands creativity, there is little use for rigid step-by-step formulae or ready-made solutions. Erickson expressed his mistrust of blind repetition when he stated, "… any theoretically based psychotherapy is mistaken because each person is different" (Zeig, 1980, p. 31). In other words, rather than relying on prefabricated responses to complex human problems, it is necessary to observe what is happening in the moment and respond with novel solutions. Even the most eloquent constructs become problematic if they do not leave room for innovation and refinement.

Any understanding of Erickson's therapy must exist as a foundation without walls. This theory of psychotherapy must capture the essence of what is being accomplished—the big picture—while freeing up the imagination for unorthodox originality. The approach of this book has been to combine a collection of case material that promotes understanding at a narrative level, with broad concepts that can lead to the development of an unlimited number of unique applications. Several overarching concepts have been introduced within the context of a unified philosophy of healing. Contained within each of these problem-solving strategies are more finite and complex descriptions of technique.

The strategies have been categorized and labeled for the purpose of conveying information in a systematic and organized manner. This does not mean that the strategies and techniques are mutually exclusive categories in which there can never be overlap. The organization of these ideas is meant to promote systematic study and professional discourse, while remaining true to the spirit of continual discovery, which characterized Erickson.

After studying hundreds of highly complex cases coming from Erickson, Short has woven together threads of continuity that can be captured using reasonably common ideas. The theoretical concepts in this text have been paired with simple analogies, folk wisdom, and illustrations from other schools of psychotherapy. One reason for this blend is to illustrate the timelessness and universal nature of these strategic principles. The information was structured in such a way as to make it easy to digest. New terminology was introduced only when it could not be avoided. In most instances, the terms employed in this text were used by Erickson. Even though he did not formally group his techniques into a class of strategies, the concepts of partitioning, progression, distraction, suggestion, reorientation, and utilization were not invented by Short but instead are drawn from Erickson's explanations of his work. The idea that several different techniques can serve the same function, and the belief that every intervention should be carried out with careful intention, also comes directly from the teaching of Milton Erickson.

This text is by no means a comprehensive summation of the clinical work of Milton Erickson: rather it is a brief introduction. One crucial component of Erickson's work that is missing from this text is the process of clinical assessment that he so skillfully applied. Each of his clinical interventions was highly individualized and could not have worked as well had there not been a systematic study of the precise dimensions of the patient's personality and life situation. Also not included in this selection is mention of Erickson's activation and dynamic use of emotional processes such as anger, vulnerability, and shock.[1] This text did not cover Erickson's use of didactic instruction, which is now commonly referred to as the psychoeducational approach. Furthermore, the

---

[1] The clinical application of these was referred to by Erickson as the "corrective emotional experience."

reader should recognize that these six strategies are not an exhaustive list. For instance, Erickson's strategic use of affective conditioning and experiential learning only received brief mention in this text.

Contraindications

Because helpful knowledge can be misapplied, common sense and good judgment should guide the implementation of each of these six strategies. As mentioned earlier in the text, partitioning should not be applied in such a way that the patient feels that the significance of his problem is being discounted or that his concerns are inconsequential. In the case of progression, the clinician should not become so distracted with breaking progress up into small steps that he overlooks immediate needs for safety or outside intervention. The strategy of reorientation is perhaps the most likely to be misapplied. It is the will of the patient, not the clinician's view, that the patient should be reoriented to. As with each of these strategies, it is foolish to act as if there were one right answer to problems, and that you have that answer. While introducing alternative perspectives for viewing reality, Erickson did not insist on one particular perspective. After pointing out numerous possibilities, he was always ready to accept any new orientation that the patient found to be useful or rewarding. For each person the "right view" is one which represents a new reality that produces hope or the appreciation of goodness in life.

The strategies of utilization and suggestion also have certain contraindications. Techniques that involve ordeals or paradoxical directives should not put the patient at increased risk of harm. Similarly, it is almost always inappropriate to ask the patient to do something that violates his or her moral code. Lastly, it is wrong to draw attention to the patient's behavior in such a way that he believes he is being mocked. To sum this all up, the patient should always be treated with dignity and respect. The primary responsibility of the clinician is to make certain that during the course of therapy no harm is done. As stated by Erickson, "All interventions should be oriented around the needs of the patient. Not the practitioner's interests or needs. Therefore, the patient is able to have

complete trust and confidence in the intentions of the practitioner"
(Erickson, 1955a).

Putting the knowledge to use

Much of the information in this book should find its way into practice through the subtle process of commonsense reasoning. The
techniques you develop to achieve a particular strategy should not
seem strange or fantastic but instead should seem natural. After
one has read about Erickson's extraordinarily creative interventions there is the temptation to attempt to replicate his work by
conjuring up fantastic and unusual therapeutic directives.
However, if the procedure seems fantastic and unusual to the therapist, there is reason to worry. Even more problematic is the temptation to directly imitate Erickson's work without having the
benefit of his unique set of skills, and without having the specific
patient to whom he tailored the intervention, and without the benefit of living in the same time period or geographical location in
which the intervention originally took place.

While seeking to develop techniques to meet the individual needs
of patients, there should be a strong sense that this procedure is
simply a reasonable thing to do. For example, if the patient has a
poor self-image and does not like to look at herself in the mirror,
then the reasonable thing to do is to help her find a way to discover her preciousness while living in the body she has been
given. But how do you accomplish this? Because she is not able to
suddenly have happy positive thoughts about herself while looking in the mirror, it makes perfect sense to break up the task by *partitioning* it into different moments in time. This provides three
options: past, present, and future. At one time she was a sweet
innocent little girl. This was before the sexual abuse by her father.
Therefore it makes perfect sense to start in the past, before the
abuse. There is some psychological distance between the past and
the here and now, thereby making it less of a threat. Having
learned that she has a photo album, which she values, it is only
reasonable to start there. While looking at herself in those photos
she begins the process of recognizing her preciousness, during that
period in time. Once this is accomplished, the strategy of *progression* can be used to help her gradually start to recognize her

preciousness in the present and eventually on into the distant future. If she were to come to a later session with her hair dyed, then a logical question to ask would be, "Do you like your new hairstyle? How does it look to you in the mirror?" When the patient indicates that she likes her new style, then this behavior is *utilized* and identified as being an important sign of progress, an indication that she feels more control over her body and the way in which she perceives it. This type of recognition will of course inspire greater hope and help her feel good about herself and her choices. For the clinician, the intervention does not seem fantastic. It simply makes sense.

All problem solving begins with the idea that change is possible. As Erickson observed, when you are dealing with someone's *life* they want you to have all the answers. Yet not everything that goes wrong can be made right. That is why it is always good to have sight of at least one small thing that can be achieved. Even the smallest breakthrough can serve as a foundation upon which other accomplishments are built. While it is not possible to cure every sickness, there is always some good that can be done for those who suffer. Even the problems that have endured for decades and baffled numerous other professionals can have a surprisingly simple solution once the emphasis is shifted to the patient's unrecognized capacity to discover an appropriate solution. When a patient lacks the confidence needed to change, it might be helpful to focus on something new, something more interesting than the problem. This creates space for unintentional progress, which can be more powerful than self-sabotage. This is all done without trying to *make* a person change. Such a position only encourages animosity. Instead, a skillful therapist knows how to foster hope and encourage resiliency so that the inner resources of the patient produce wellbeing.

"When you read a book backwards ... you read a different book
than if you read it first chapter to last ... You should read
a good book backwards, start with the last chapter, then
read the second to last chapter and so on.
After you have done so, reread it front to back
and you will have a marvelous experience."
—Milton H. Erickson, August 6, 1974

Appendix A

Self-Development Exercises

The strategies described in this book can yield powerful results when put into action by a competent practitioner. As Erickson would sometimes say of hypnosis, the best way to learn about it is to experience it directly. In order to use these six strategies competently, it is highly recommended that a good amount of time and thought be invested in an analysis of relevant personal experiences. These may be memorable experiences from your past or yet undiscovered opportunities for personal growth.

It is one thing to act as an outside observer and watch others solve important life challenges. But an effort to vigorously seek out opportunities to apply problem-solving strategies to one's own life produces a much richer return. It is this spirit of ongoing personal development that adds authenticity to one's efforts. If you are not certain how to structure this task on your own, then what follow are some thought experiments that have been designed to illustrate each of the different strategies.

Distraction

In order to promote an experiential understanding of the preceding material, an exercise has been developed with distraction as the core feature. It should be noted that distraction is not an easy strategy to perform on oneself. In order to be truly distracted a person would need to be *not* thinking about what he or she is planning to do. Of course there are those who frequently distract themselves by turning to excessive work, addiction to entertainment, sex, or drugs. Each of these can provide an effective distraction from painful realities. However, these do not provide the same clinical benefit as the more short-lived method of distraction that strategically moves the individual toward a new recognition of personal ability.

Exercise

Meditate on the following words: "sex," "control," "love," "power," "beauty."

Step 1: Think about a time in the past when you have been so thoroughly distracted by something that your actions became automatic. What was it that was so distracting and why did it gain control of your attention?

Step 2: Spend some time thinking about all of the things you were able to accomplish without paying attention to what you were doing. This is similar to the experience of driving yourself to a familiar destination without stopping to think where you are going or what your hands and feet are doing. Hopefully, you will think of an event that has personal meaning. You should focus on behaviors that you might have been too inhibited to attempt had you not been so thoroughly distracted.

Step 3: Lock the memory of this event into consciousness. During the next several days return to this memory as often as possible. The passing of time will be an important part of this exercise in distraction.

Step 4: Do not expect immediate results. After two or three weeks have passed, spend some time reviewing your actions since first reading these instructions.

Partitioning

One of the best ways to understand the role of partitioning in human problem solving is to experience its effect first-hand. Hopefully, while reading the text, you have stopped to consider times in your life when you felt better able to deal with a problem once it was broken down into smaller parts. It may even be that you have already incorporated this in your therapy without realizing that it is a clinical strategy with broad applications.

In order to promote an experiential understanding of the preceding material, an exercise has been developed with partitioning as the core feature. Although this exercise has been designed as a learning exercise for professionals, some practitioners have used the same procedure in their clinical practice with good results.

Exercise

Step 1: Think about a time when you felt overwhelmed by life circumstances. Think about all the different factors that contributed to an overall feeling of distress. If there is a painful or traumatic memory that might be brought up by this exercise, then take a few moments to make certain you are ready to do this sort of deep work.

Step 2: Now visualize a brick wall in front of you. The brick wall represents the barrier standing between you and happiness. If you are a tactile learner, then you can actually construct a barrier using small objects that are lined up like a wall. Each brick in this wall represents some aspect of the problem. Take a few minutes to put names to the various pieces of the problem.

Step 3: Spend some time focusing on your desire to cross this barrier. You no longer want to be stuck on the distressing side of the problem. To achieve peace and comfort you must get through to that space on the other side. You will feel much better once you can get over there.

Step 4: Now focus your attention on the part of the problem that you are best prepared to deal with at this time. Focus on a single brick and think about what you could do or say that would allow you to knock it out of your way. (If you are using a physical wall, then you can move aside one of the objects once you have successfully dealt with it.)

Step 5: Now focus your attention on a part of the problem that you have experienced sometime in the past, and successfully overcome. This should allow you to knock some more bricks from the wall.

Step 6: Now think about a part of the problem you could find support for. Spend some time thinking about various small ways that others would be willing to help you out.

Step 7: The wall can be further fragmented by considering which part of the problem is least concerning to you. Think about which aspects of the problem you could comfortably live with for now.

Step 8: Ask yourself which part of the problem is most likely to change with time. Which of these issues might resolve themselves without any effort on your part? This will allow you to knock out several more bricks.

Step 9: If you have created enough space to pass through, then you can visualize yourself walking through to the other side. Circle around the remaining parts of the wall. Decide whether you are ready to stop here or want to find other ways that you can devise to further fragment the problem.

Note: For the purposes of this book, this exercise has been scripted for use by a single individual. However, the exercise can also be used in a group setting. The wall is constructed using a line of people who have their arms linked together. The person who must get through the wall identifies each individual as some piece of the problem. Once that part of the problem is dealt with, the arms are unlinked or the individual might be asked to return to their seat. Once the work is complete, the person will have the opportunity to physically walk through the wall. This often produces powerful results, with visible changes in the demeanor of the individual.

Progression

In order to promote an experiential understanding of the preceding material, an exercise has been developed with progression as the core feature. As with all of the techniques found in this book, it is not necessary to follow the exercise in a rigid manner. If there are some ways you would like to modify this exercise to meet your personal needs, then you should do so.

Exercise

Step 1: Think about something you wish you could accomplish but do not feel able. Reach deep inside. It is best to find something that seems so out of reach that you have not allowed yourself to consider it as an option.

Step 2: Take a sheet of paper and write the following sentence at the *bottom* of the page: "My hope is that someday I will be able to _____" [fill in the blank].

Step 3: Now, at the *top* of the page, for #1, write down the main reason why this has not seemed possible for you. Then finish the following sentence: "This excuse for not making progress is not entirely correct because _____" [fill in the blank].

Step 4: For #2, write down the smallest, simplest thing you could do that would point you in the direction of the accomplishment you have listed at the bottom of the page. This is just one, very small step forward.

Step 5: For #3, think about what you have listed at the bottom of the page and how it can be broken down into several smaller components. List three or four of these component actions that have occurred in the past, perhaps by accident. Now list the number of days that might go by before you accidentally repeat one of the component skills.

Step 6: Spend five or more minutes visualizing yourself doing the thing that you have listed at the bottom of the page. Watch yourself from the eyes of an outside observer. Do not stop the meditation until you are satisfied with the image you achieve.

Step 7: For #4, list the names of all the people who would be willing to encourage or support you in your effort to achieve this goal.

Step 8: For #5, list any other small steps that you can think of that would eventually bring you further toward the final goal. After the last step, draw an arrow pointing down toward the goal at the bottom of the page. This is symbolic of your gradual progression in that direction.

Suggestion

The exercise listed below will perhaps seem to be the most simplistic of the exercises but it is not something to be quickly dismissed. The results can be surprising and the willingness to commit this type of energy to one's personal goals is in itself a worthy endeavor.

Exercise

Step 1: While in bed, check to make certain that you can see the time on a bedside clock. After noting what time it is, pick a specific time when you would like to awaken. For instance, 6:50 a.m., ten minutes before the alarm normally awakens you.

Step 2: With your eyes closed, repeat silently to yourself, "Wake me up at 6:50, wake me up at 6:50, wake me up at 6:50 …" You should say this at least 100 times or until you fall asleep. (For some folks, this exercise has the additional benefit of putting them to sleep more quickly than usual.) Unless your unconscious mind has some good reason for foiling your plans, you should wake up at the appointed time.

Step 3: Now that you have some confidence in the method and the outcome, pick a more personally meaningful goal. For instance, "I will be more assertive with my in-laws, I will be more assertive with my in-laws …" This is something you should do each night for a period of two weeks. Make certain to pick a goal in which there is a realistic chance for improvement while at the same time interesting enough to keep you from becoming bored with the task.

Step 4: Watch for smalls signs indicating progress. Allowing yourself to develop some new positive expectancies is just as important as the repetition of the direction suggestion.

Reorientation

In order to promote an experiential understanding of the preceding material, an exercise has been developed with reorientation as the core feature. As with all of the techniques found in this book, it is not necessary to follow the exercise in a rigid manner. This exercise is the type that can be practiced while you are driving home from work. If you were to apply this strategy to your work as a clinician, there is no doubt that you would derive great personal benefit.

Exercise

Step 1: Think of a problem that you have seen in one of your patients and the solution or intervention that you suggested. From all of your therapeutic interactions during the day, pick the one that interests you the most.

Step 2: Carefully consider the essential features of their problem. View it as something on a continuum that can exist to a greater or lesser degree. Next, locate your own behavior or emotional experiences somewhere on that continuum. For instance, if you have a patient who has become angry and punched his wife in the face, then move down the continuum a little way to a time when you felt angry at your spouse and said something hurtful. In other words, explore your own subjective understanding of what it is to have this type of problematic urge.

Step 3: Remind yourself of the intervention that took place during therapy. Pay careful attention to the most important statements you made while helping this person deal with their problem. What did you tell the patient to say or do? What kind of thinking did you want the patient to accomplish? Whatever it was, take the intervention and adapt it to your life situation as well as possible. If you wanted your patient to think about how his wife felt after being punched in the face, then think about how your spouse felt after hearing what you had to say during the last argument. In this way, you are not asking someone to do something that you are not willing to try yourself.

Step 4: Pay careful attention to what it feels like to be the subject of your therapy. Meditate on the new insights you have achieved.

Lastly, strive to be one of your least resistant patients. Practice this exercise as much as you can find time to do. This way you are more likely to benefit from your own wisdom and experience.

Utilization

In order to promote an experiential understanding of the preceding material, an exercise has been developed with utilization as the core feature. To be successful at this exercise, one simply needs to develop a new awareness of personal skills and/or situational possibilities that exist as untapped resources. When this occurs the experience is most gratifying.

Exercise

Step 1: First, decide what you want to utilize. This can be some aspect of your personality, events that are occurring around you, or mistakes that have been made by you or others. Think of something that is not easily altered or undone. Examine situations in which you have invested a good deal of energy resisting. Write down on a piece of paper this thing that you have not been able to control and therefore might as well utilize.

Step 2: Next, write the following sentence: "This would have been acceptable if only it had led to _____" [fill in the blank].

Step 3: Utilization requires an attitude of acceptance. Think about the thing that you listed in Step 1. Look at it from a perspective that allows for some humor. A person cannot take him/herself too seriously and still have the attitude of acceptance necessary for utilization. Write the following sentence: "It would be really funny if I _____" [fill in the blank].

Step 4: Give yourself time for insights to occur. There is more than one way to utilize each event or behavior. After you have had some time to meditate, complete the following sentence: "Because of _____ it is now possible for me to _____" [the first blank is filled in with what you listed in Step 1; the second blank is up to your imagination].

Step 5: Develop a plan for how you can implement insights from Step 4. Outline your utilization experiment. If things do not turn out as you planned, then look for a way to utilize the failure. Make it a valuable learning experience that leads to other opportunities for growth.

References

Arlow, J. A. (1989), "Psychoanalysis," in R. J. Corsini and D. Wedding (eds), *Current Psychotherapies*, 4th edn (Itasca, Illinois: F. E. Peacock).

Baker, M. (2004), *A Tribute to Elizabeth Moore Erickson: Colleague Extraordinaire, Wife, Mother, and Companion* (Mexico City: Alom Editores).

Bandura, A. (2003), "On shaping one's future: The exercise of personal agency," keynote Address at the Milton H. Erickson Foundation Brief Therapy Conference, San Francisco, December 12, 2003.

Bateson, G. (1972), *Steps to an Ecology of Mind* (New York, NY: Ballantine).

Battino, R., and South, T. L. (2005), *Ericksonian Approaches: A Comprehensive Manual*, 2nd edn (Carmarthen, UK: Crown House Publishing).

Beaulieu, D. (2002), "Talk to Your Patient's Eyes Not Just Their Ear!," audio recording of the Brief Therapy Conference, Orlando, Florida, December 12–15 (Phoenix, AZ: Milton H. Erickson Foundation, Phoenix, AZ).

Beavers, W. R. (1985), *Successful Marriage: A Family Systems Approach to Couples Therapy* (New York, NY: W. W. Norton & Co.).

Beecher, H. K. (1961), "Surgery as placebo: A quantitative study of bias," *Journal of the American Medical Association, 176*, pp. 1102–7.

Bornstein, R. F. (1989), "Exposure and affect: Overview and meta-analysis of research, 1968–1987," *Psychological Bulletin, 106*, pp. 265–89.

Carlson, N. R. (2004), *Physiology of Behavior*, 8th edn (New York, NY: Allan & Bacon).

Cialdini, R. B. (1995), "Principles and techniques of social influence," in A. Tesser (ed.), *Advanced Social Psychology* (New York, NY: McGraw-Hill), (pp. 257–81).

Clark, D. M. (1986), "A cognitive approach to panic," *Behavior Research and Treatment, 24*, pp. 461–71.

Connolly, T., et al. (1995), *The Well-Managed Classroom: Promoting Student Success Through Social Skill Instruction* (Boys Town, NB: Boys Town Press.

Council, J. R. (1999), "Hypnosis and response expectancies," in I. Kirsch (ed.), *How Expectancies Shape Experience* (Washington, D.C.: American Psychological Association) pp. 383–402.

Cummings, N. A., and Cummings, J. L. (2000), *The Essence of Psychotherapy: Reinventing the Art in the New Era of Data* (New York, NY: Academic Press).

De Shazer, S. (1994), *Words Were Originally Magic* (New York, NY: W. W. Norton & Co.).

De Shazer, S., and Berg, I. K. (1997), "An Interview by Dan Short with Steve de Shazer and Insoo Kim Berg," *Milton H Erickson Foundation Newsletter*, 17, 2 (Phoenix, AZ: Milton H. Erickson Foundation Archives), p. 1.

Dolan, Y. (2000), an interview with Yvonne Dolan, MSW, by Dan Short, *Milton H. Erickson Foundation Newsletter*, 20, 2 (Phoenix, AZ: Milton H. Erickson Foundation Archives).

Duncan, B. L., Miller, S. D., and Sparks, J. A. (2004). *The Heroic Client: A Revolutionary Way to Improve Effectiveness Through Client-Directed, Outcome-Informed Therapy*, (San Francisco, CA: Jossey-Bass).

Ekman, P. (1992), *Telling Lies: Clues to Deceit in the Marketplace, Politics, and Marriage* (New York, NY: W.W. Norton & Co.).

Erickson, M. H. (c. 1930/2001), "Posthypnotic Suggestion for Ejaculatio Praecox," previously unpublished manuscript, in *Milton H. Erickson M.D.: The Complete Works* (digital media published by the Milton H. Erickson Foundation).

Erickson, M. H. (1936/2001), "Migraine Headache in a Resistant Patient." previously unpublished manuscript, in *Milton H. Erickson M.D.: The Complete Works* (digital media published by the Milton H. Erickson Foundation).

Erickson, M. H. (1939/2001), "Applications of hypnosis to psychiatry," *Medical Record*, July 19, pp. 60–5 (originally from an address given before the Ontario Neuropsychiatric Association, March 18, 1937, at London, Ontario), in *Milton H. Erickson M.D.: The Complete Works* (digital media published by the Milton H. Erickson Foundation).

Erickson, M. H. (1940/2001), "Appearance in Three Generations of an Atypical Pattern of the Sneezing Reflex," *The Journal of Genetic Psychology*, 56, pp. 455–9, in *Milton H. Erickson M.D.: The Complete Works* (digital media published by the Milton H. Erickson Foundation).

Erickson, M. H. (1941/2001a), "The Early Recognition of Mental Disease" speech, April 24, 1940, at the Post-Graduate Clinic for General Practitioners, Eloise Hospital, Eloise, Michigan, published in *Diseases of the Nervous System* (March), in *Milton H. Erickson M.D.: The Complete Works* (digital media published by the Milton H. Erickson Foundation).

Erickson, M. H. (1941/2001b), "Hypnosis: A general review," *Diseases of the Nervous System*, January, pp. 1–8, in *Milton H. Erickson M.D.: The Complete Works* (digital media published by the Milton H. Erickson Foundation).

Erickson, M. H. (1948/2001), "Hypnotic Psychotherapy," The Medical Clinics of North America, May 1948, in *Milton H. Erickson M.D.: The Complete Works* (digital media published by the Milton H. Erickson Foundation).

Erickson, M. H. (1952), a lecture by Milton H. Erickson, Los Angeles, June 25, Audio Recording No. CD/EMH.52.6.25 (Phoenix, AZ: Milton H. Erickson Foundation Archives).

Erickson, M. H. (1952/2001a), "A therapeutic double bind utilizing resistance," unpublished manuscript, in *Milton H. Erickson M.D.: The Complete Works* (digital media published by the Milton H. Erickson Foundation).

Erickson, M. H. (1952/2001b), "Deep Hypnosis and Its Induction," in *Milton H. Erickson M.D.: The Complete Works* (digital media published by the Milton H. Erickson Foundation).

Erickson, M. H. (1954/2001), "A Clinical Note on Indirect Hypnotic Therapy," *Journal of Clinical and Experimental Hypnosis*, 2, pp. 171–74), in *Milton H. Erickson M.D.: The Complete Works* (digital media published by the Milton H. Erickson Foundation).

Erickson, M. H. (1955a), a lecture by Milton H. Erickson, Philadelphia, August, Audio Recording No. CD/EMH.55.8 (Phoenix, AZ: Milton H. Erickson Foundation Archives).

Erickson, M. H. (1955b), a lecture by Milton H. Erickson, Boston, September 29, Audio Recording No. CD/EMH.55.9.29 (Phoenix, AZ: Milton H. Erickson Foundation Archives).

Erickson, M. H. (1955/2001), "Self-Exploration in the Hypnotic State," *Journal of Clinical and Experimental Hypnosis*, 3, pp. 49–57, in *Milton H. Erickson M.D.: The Complete Works* (digital media published by the Milton H. Erickson Foundation).

Erickson, M. H. (1956), a lecture by Milton H. Erickson, Phoenix, June, Audio Recording No. CD/EMH.56.6 (Phoenix, AZ: Milton H. Erickson Foundation Archives).

Erickson, M. H. (1957), a lecture by Milton H. Erickson, Los Angeles, October 19, Audio Recording No. CD/EMH.57.10.19 (Phoenix, AZ: Milton H. Erickson Foundation Archives).

Erickson, M. H. (1958a), a lecture by Milton H. Erickson, San Diego, February 23 Audio Recording No. CD/EMH.58.2.23 (Phoenix, AZ: Milton H. Erickson Foundation Archives).

Erickson, M. H. (1958b), a lecture by Milton H. Erickson, Chicago, October 1, Audio Recording No. CD/EMH.58.10.1 (Phoenix, AZ: Milton H. Erickson Foundation Archives).

Erickson, M. H. (1958c), a lecture by Milton H. Erickson, Pasadena, October 31 Audio Recording No. CD/EMH.58.10.31 (Phoenix, AZ: Milton H. Erickson Foundation Archives).

Erickson, M. H. (1958d), a lecture by Milton H. Erickson, Philadelphia, November 11, Audio Recording No. CD/EMH.58.11.11 (Phoenix, AZ: Milton H. Erickson Foundation Archives).

Erickson, M. H. (1958e), a lecture by Milton H. Erickson, Philadelphia, November 12, Audio Recording No. CD/EMH.58.11.12 (Phoenix, AZ: Milton H. Erickson Foundation Archives).

Erickson, M. H. (1958f), a lecture by Milton H. Erickson, Palo Alto, November 24, Audio Recording No. CD/EMH.58.11.24 (Phoenix, AZ: Milton H. Erickson Foundation Archives).

Erickson, M. H. (1958g), "Deep Hypnosis and Its Induction," in L. M. Le Cron (ed.), *Experimental Hypnosis* (New York, NY: Macmillan Company) pp. 70–112.

Erickson, M. H. (1958/2001), "Pediatric Hypnotherapy," *American Journal of Clinical Hypnosis 1*, pp. 25–9, in *Milton H. Erickson M.D.: The Complete Works* (digital media published by the Milton H. Erickson Foundation).

Erickson, M. H. (1959a), lecture by Milton H. Erickson, Utica, NY, February 14, Audio Recording No. CD/EMH.59.2.14 (Phoenix, AZ: Milton H. Erickson Foundation Archives).

Erickson, M. H. (1959b), a lecture by Milton H. Erickson, Boston, June 19, Audio Recording No. CD/EMH.59.6.19 (Phoenix, AZ: Milton H. Erickson Foundation Archives).

Erickson, M. H. (1959c), a lecture by Milton H. Erickson, San Francisco, September 11, Audio Recording No. CD/EMH.59.9.11 (Phoenix, AZ: Milton H. Erickson Foundation Archives).

Erickson, M. H. (1959d), a lecture by Milton H. Erickson, Phoenix, November 15, Audio Recording No. CD/EMH.59.11.15 (Phoenix, AZ: Milton H. Erickson Foundation Archives).

Erickson, M. H. (1959/2001), "Further Clinical Techniques of Hypnosis: Utilization Techniques," *American Journal of Clinical Hypnosis*, 2, pp. 3–21, in *Milton H. Erickson M.D.: The Complete Works* (digital media published by the Milton H. Erickson Foundation.)

Erickson, M. H. (1960a), a lecture by Milton H. Erickson, Boston, March 21, Audio Recording No. CD/EMH.60.3.21 (Phoenix, AZ: Milton H. Erickson Foundation Archives).

Erickson, M. H. (1960b), a lecture by Milton H. Erickson, Chicago, June 10, Audio Recording No. CD/EMH.60.6.10 (Phoenix, AZ: Milton H. Erickson Foundation Archives).

Erickson, M. H. (1960c), a lecture by Milton H. Erickson, Miami, August 3, Audio Recording No. CD/EMH.60.8.3 (Phoenix, AZ: Milton H. Erickson Foundation Archives).

Erickson, M. H. (1961a), a lecture by Milton H. Erickson, Stanford, May 27, Audio Recording No. CD/EMH.61.5.27 (Phoenix, AZ: Milton H. Erickson Foundation Archives).

Erickson, M. H. (1961b), a lecture by Milton H. Erickson, San Diego, July 22, Audio Recording No. CD/EMH.61.7.22 (Phoenix, AZ: Milton H. Erickson Foundation Archives).

Erickson, M. H. (1961/2001a), "Definition of Hypnosis," *Encyclopaedia Britannica*, 14th edn, in *Milton H. Erickson M.D.: The Complete Works* (digital media published by the Milton H. Erickson Foundation).

Erickson, M. H. (1961/2001b), "Historical note on the hand levitation and other ideomotor techniques," *American Journal of Clinical Hypnosis*, 3, pp. 196–9, in *Milton H. Erickson M.D.: The Complete Works* (digital media published by the Milton H. Erickson Foundation).

Erickson, M. H. (1962a), a lecture by Milton H. Erickson, San Diego, April 29, Audio Recording No. CD/EMH.62.4.29 (Phoenix, AZ: Milton H. Erickson Foundation Archives).

Erickson, M. H. (1962b), a lecture by Milton H. Erickson, Calgary, Canada, June 18, Audio Recording No. CD/EMH.62.6.18 (Phoenix, AZ: Milton H. Erickson Foundation Archives).

Erickson, M. H. (1962c), a lecture by Milton H. Erickson, Los Angeles, October 10, Audio Recording No. CD/EMH.62.10.27 (Phoenix, AZ: Milton H. Erickson Foundation Archives).

Erickson, M. H. (1962d), a lecture by Milton H. Erickson, Chicago, October 17, Audio Recording No. CD/EMH.62.10.17 (Phoenix, AZ: Milton H. Erickson Foundation Archives).

Erickson, M. H. (1962/2001), an audio recording for the ASCH 1962 series on Hypnotic Induction, in *Milton H. Erickson M.D.: The Complete Works* (digital media published by the Milton H. Erickson Foundation).

Erickson, M. H. (1963), a lecture by Milton H. Erickson, San Diego, April 4, Audio Recording No. CD/EMH.63.4.4 (Phoenix, AZ: Milton H. Erickson Foundation Archives).

Erickson, M. H. (1964a), a lecture by Milton H. Erickson, Chicago, March 6, Audio Recording No. CD/EMH.64.3.6 (Phoenix, AZ: Milton H. Erickson Foundation Archives).

Erickson, M. H. (1964b), a lecture by Milton H. Erickson, Boston, December, Audio Recording No. CD/EMH.64.12 (Phoenix, AZ: Milton H. Erickson Foundation Archives).

Erickson, M. H. (1964/2001a), "The Burden of Responsibility in Effective Psychotherapy," *American Journal of Clinical Hypnosis*, 6, pp. 269–71, in *Milton H. Erickson M.D.: The Complete Works* (digital media published by the Milton H. Erickson Foundation).

Erickson, M. H. (1964/2001b), "A Hypnotic Technique for Resistant Patients: The Patient, the Technique, and its Rationale, and Field Experiments," *American Journal of Clinical Hypnosis 7*, pp. 8–32, in *Milton H. Erickson M.D.: The Complete Works* (digital media published by the Milton H. Erickson Foundation).

Erickson, M. H. (1964/2001c), "Initial Experiments Investigating the Nature of Hypnosis," *American Journal of Clinical Hypnosis*, 7, pp. 152–62, in *Milton H. Erickson M.D.: The Complete Works* (digital media published by the Milton H. Erickson Foundation).

Erickson, M. H. (1964/2001d), "The Confusion Technique in Hypnosis," *American Journal of Clinical Hypnosis*, January, 1964, 6, pp. 183–207, in *Milton H. Erickson M.D.: The Complete Works* (digital media published by the Milton H. Erickson Foundation).

Erickson, M. H. (1965a), a lecture by Milton H. Erickson, Phoenix, January 25, Audio Recording No. CD/EMH.65.1.25 (Phoenix, AZ: Milton H. Erickson Foundation Archives).

Erickson, M. H. (1965b), a lecture by Milton H. Erickson, Seattle, May 21, Audio Recording No. CD/EMH.65.5.21 (Phoenix, AZ: Milton H. Erickson Foundation Archives).

Erickson, M. H. (1965c), a lecture by Milton H. Erickson, San Francisco, July 16, Audio Recording No. CD/EMH.65.7.16 (Phoenix, AZ: Milton H. Erickson Foundation Archives).

Erickson, M. H. (1966), a lecture by Milton H. Erickson, Houston, February 18, Audio Recording No. CD/EMH.66.2.18 (Phoenix, AZ: Milton H. Erickson Foundation Archives).

Erickson, M. H. (1966/2001), "The Interspersal Hypnotic Technique for Symptom Correction and Pain Control," in *Milton H. Erickson M.D.: The Complete Works* (digital media published by the Milton H. Erickson Foundation).

Erickson, M. H. (1967), a lecture by Milton H. Erickson, Delaware, September 19, Audio Recording No. CD/EMH.67.9.19 (Phoenix, AZ: Milton H. Erickson Foundation Archives).

Erickson, M. H. (1973/2001a), "Literalness and the Use of Trance in Neurosis. Dialogue between Milton H. Erickson and Ernest L. Rossi, 1973," in *Milton H. Erickson M.D.: The Complete Works* (digital media published by the Milton H. Erickson Foundation).

Erickson, M. H. (1973/2001b), "A Field Investigation by Hypnosis of Sound Loci Importance in Human Behavior," *American Journal of Clinical Hypnosis*, 16, pp 147–64, in *Milton H. Erickson M.D.: The Complete Works* (digital media published by the Milton H. Erickson Foundation).

Erickson, M. H. (1977a), a teaching seminar by Milton H. Erickson, Phoenix, June, Audio Recording No. CD/EMH.77.6 (Phoenix, AZ: Milton H. Erickson Foundation Archives).

Erickson, M. H. (1977b), a teaching seminar by Milton H. Erickson, Phoenix, November, Audio Recording No. CD/EMH.77.11.a (Phoenix, AZ: Milton H. Erickson Foundation Archives).

Erickson, M. H. (1977/2001), "Hypnotic Approaches to Therapy," *American Journal of Clinical Hypnosis*, 20 (1), pp. 20–35, in *Milton H. Erickson M.D.: The Complete Works* (digital media published by the Milton H. Erickson Foundation).

Erickson, M. H. (1979), teaching seminar, Phoenix, December, Audio Recording No. CD/EMH.79.12 (Phoenix, AZ: Milton H. Erickson Foundation Archives).

Erickson, M. H. (1980a), teaching seminar, Phoenix, February 14, Audio Recording No. CD/EMH.80.2.14 (Phoenix, AZ: Milton H. Erickson Foundation Archives).

Erickson, M. H. (1980b), teaching seminar, Phoenix, February 12, Audio Recording No. CD/EMH.80.2.12 (Phoenix, AZ: Milton H. Erickson Foundation Archives).

Erickson, M. H. (1983), *Healing in Hypnosis*, ed. E. L. Rossi, M. O. Ryan, and F. A. Sharp, (New York, NY: Irvington).

Erickson, M. H., Hershman, S., and Sector, I. I. (1961), *The Practical Application of Medical and Dental Hypnosis* (New York, NY: Julian Press).

Erickson, M. H., and Kubie, L. (1938/2001), "The use of automatic drawing in the interpretation and relief of a state of acute obsessional depression," *Psychoanalytic Quarterly*, 7, 4, in *Milton H. Erickson M.D.: The Complete Works* (digital media published by the Milton H. Erickson Foundation).

Erickson, M. H., and Rossi, E. L. (1979), *Hypnotherapy: An Exploratory Casebook* (New York, NY: Irvington Publishers).

Erickson, M. H., and Rossi, E. L. (1981), *Experiencing Hypnosis: Therapeutic Approaches to Altered States* (New York, NY: Irvington Publishers).

Erickson, M. H., Rossi, E. L., and Rossi, S. I. (1976), *Hypnotic Realities: The Induction of Clinical Hypnosis and Forms of Indirect Suggestion* (New York, NY: Irvington Publishers).

Erickson, M. H., Rossi, E. L., and Rossi, S. I. (1976/2001), "Milton H. Erickson's Approaches to Trance Induction," paper presented at the 28th annual meeting of the Society for Clinical and Experimental Hypnosis, in *Milton H. Erickson M.D.: The Complete Works* (digital media published by the Milton H. Erickson Foundation).

Erickson, M. H., and Zeig, J. K. (1977/2001), "Symptom prescription for expanding the psychotic's world view," paper presented by J. K. Zeig to the 20th Annual Scientific Meeting of the American Society of Clinical Hypnosis, October 20, Atlanta, Georgia, in *Milton H. Erickson M.D.: The Complete Works* (digital media published by the Milton H. Erickson Foundation).

Erickson-Elliott, B. A., and Erickson-Klein, R. (1991), "Milton H. Erickson's Increasing Shift to Less Directive Hypnotic Techniques as Illustrated by Work with Family Members," in S. R. Lankton, S. G. Gilligan, and J. K. Zeig (eds), *Ericksonian Monographs*, No. 8 (New York, NY: Brunner/Mazel).

Erickson-Klein, R. (1990), "Pain Control Interventions of Milton H. Erickson," in J. K. Zeig and S. Gilligan (eds), *Brief Therapy* (New York, NY: Brunner/Mazel), (pp. 273–87).

Ewin, D. (1996), Dabney Ewin, MD (an interview by J. Parsons-Fein), *Milton H. Erickson Foundation Newsletter*, *16*, 2, Milton H. Erickson Foundation Archives, Phoenix, AZ, pp. 1, 18–20.

Fazio, R. H., and Zanna, M. P. (1981), "Direct experience and attitude behavior consistency," in L. Berkowitz (ed.), *Advances in Experimental Social Psychology*, Vol. 14 (New York, NY: Academic Press) pp. 161–202.

Finn, S. E., and Tonsager, M. E. (1997), "Information-gathering and therapeutic models of assessment: complementary paradigms," *Psychological Assessment*, *9*, pp. 374–85.

Fish, J. M. (1973), *Placebo Therapy* (San Francisco: Jossey-Bass).

Frank, J. D. (1973), *Persuasion and Healing*, rev. edn, (Baltimore, MD: Johns Hopkins University Press).

Frankl, V. E. (1939), "Zur medikamentösen unterstützung der psychotherapie bei neurosen," *Schweizer Archiv für Neurologie und Psychiatrie*, *43*, pp. 26–31.

Frankl, V. E. (1973), *The Doctor and the Soul* (New York, NY: Vintage Books).

Frankl, V. E. (1977), *The Unheard Cry for Meaning: Psychotherapy and Humanism* (New York, NY: Simon and Schuster).

Frankl, V. E. (1984), *Man's Search for Meaning: An Introduction to Logotherapy* (New York, NY: Simon & Schuster).

Frankl, V. E. (1996), an Interview with Viktor Frankl, MD, by Dan Short, *Milton H. Erickson Foundation Newsletter*, *16*, 3 (Phoenix, AZ: Milton H. Erickson Foundation Archives).

Freedman, J. L., and Fraser, S. C. (1966), "Compliance without pressure: The foot-in-the-door technique," *Journal of Personality and Social Psychology*, *4*, pp. 195–203.

Freud, S. (1912/1966), *The Basic Writings of Sigmund Freud* (New York, NY: Modern Library).

Gardner, G. (1974), "Hypnosis with children," *International Journal of Clinical and Experimental Hypnosis, 22*, pp. 20–38.

Gilligan, S. (1987), *Therapeutic Trances: The Cooperation Principle in Ericksonian Hypnotherapy* (New York, NY: Brunner/Mazel).

Gilligan, S. (2001), "Getting to the core," *Family Therapy Networker*, January/February, pp. 22–9, 54–5.

Gordon, D., and Myers-Anderson, M. (1981), *Phoenix: Therapeutic Patterns of Milton H. Erickson, M.D.* (Cupertino, California: Meta).

Haley, J. (1973), *Uncommon Therapy: The Psychiatric Techniques of Milton H. Erickson, M.D.* (New York, NY: W. W. Norton & Co.).

Haley, J. (1984), *Ordeal Therapy: Unusual Ways to Change Behavior* (San Francisco: Jossey-Bass).

Haley, J. (1985), *Conversations with Milton H. Erickson, M.D., Volumes I-III* (New York, NY: Triangle Press).

Honigfeld, G. (1964), "Non-specific factors in treatment: I. Review of placebo reactions and placebo reactors," *Diseases of the Nervous System, 25*, pp. 145–56.

Horvath, A. O., and Symonds, B. D. (1991), "Relation between working alliance and outcome in psychotherapy: A meta-analysis," *Journal of Counseling Psychology, 38*, 139–49.

Horwitz, A. V. (1982), *The Social Control of Mental Illness: Studies on Law and Social Control* (New York, NY: Academic Press).

Howard, D. J. (1990), "The influence of verbal responses to common greetings on compliance behavior: The foot-in-the-mouth effect," *Journal of Applied Social Psychology, 20*, pp. 1185–96.

Hubble, M. A., Duncan, B. L., and Miller, S. D. (1999), "Directing attention to what works," in M.A. Hubble, B. L. Duncan, and S. D. Miller (eds), *The Heart and Soul of Change: What Works in* Therapy (pp. 389–406, Washington, DC: American Psychological Association).

Hughes, J. C., and Rothovius, A. E. (1996), *The World's Greatest Hypnotists* (New York, NY: University Press of America).

Kirsch, I. (1990), *Changing Expectations: A Key to Effective Psychotherapy* (Pacific Grove, CA: Brooks/Cole).

Klopfer, B. (1957), "Psychological variables in human cancer," *Journal of Projective Techniques*, *21*, pp. 331–40.

Kübler-Ross, E. (1969), *On Death and Dying* (New York, NY: Macmillan).

Lankton, S. R. (1997/2003), "Milton Erickson's Contribution to Therapy: Epistemology—Not Technology," in S. R. Lankton, *Assembling Ericksonian Therapy: The Collected Papers of Stephen Lankton* (Phoenix, AZ: Zeig, Tucker, & Theisen), pp. 25–38.

Lankton, S. R. (2001/2003), "Ericksonian Therapy," in S. R. Lankton, *Assembling Ericksonian Therapy: The Collected Papers of Stephen Lankton*, (Phoenix, AZ: Zeig, Tucker, & Theisen), pp. 1–24.

Lankton, S. R., and Lankton, C. H. (1983), *The Answer Within: A Clinical Framework of Ericksonian Hypnotherapy* (New York, NY: Brunner/Mazel).

Lerner, B., and Fiske, D. W. (1973), "Patient attributes and the eye of the beholder," *Journal of Consulting and Clinical Psychology*, *40*, pp. 272–7.

Loriedo, C. (1997), interview with Camillo Loriedo by Dan Short, *Milton H. Erickson Foundation Newsletter*, *17*, 3 (Phoenix, AZ: Milton H. Erickson Foundation).

Love, P. (2003), "Neuro-Affective Therapy: Heart, Soul, Science, and Strategy," audio recording of *Three Voices*, Phoenix, Arizona, March 7–9 (Phoenix, AZ: Milton H. Erickson Foundation).

Matthews, W. J. (2000), "Ericksonian approaches to hypnosis and therapy: Where are we now?," *International Journal of Clinical and Experimental Hypnosis*, *48*, 4, pp. 418–36.

Matthews, W. J., Lankton, S., and Lankton, C. (1993), "An Ericksonian Model of Hypnotherapy," in J. W. Rhue, S. J. Lynn, and I. Kirsch (eds), *Handbook of Clinical Hypnosis* (Washington, DC: American Psychological Association).

Mischel, W. (1984), "Convergences and challenges in the search for consistency", *American Psychologist*, *39*(4), pp. 351–64.

Murphy, S. T., and Zajonc, R. B. (1993), "Affect, cognition, and awareness: Affective priming with optimal and suboptimal exposures," *Journal of Personality and Social Psychology*, *64*, pp. 723–39.

O'Hanlon, W. H. (1987), *Taproots: Underlying Principles of Milton Erickson's Therapy and Hypnosis* (New York, NY: W. W. Norton & Co.).

O'Hanlon, W. H., and Hexum, A. L. (1990), *An Uncommon Casebook: The Complete Clinical Work of Milton H. Erickson, M.D.* (New York, NY: W. W. Norton & Co.).

Obermiller, C. (1985), "Varieties of mere exposure: The effects of processing style and repetition on affective response." *Journal of Consumer Research*, 12, pp. 17–30.

Olness, K., Culbert, T., and Uden, D. (1989), "Self-regulation of salivary immunoglobulin A by children," *Pediatrics*, 83, pp. 66–71.

Orlinsky, D. E., Grawe, K., and Parks, B. K. (1994), "Process and outcome in psychotherapy—noch einmal," in A. E. Bergin and S. L. Garfield (eds), *Handbook of Psychotherapy and Behavior Change*, 4th edn, pp. 270–378 (New York, NY: Wiley).

Orlinsky, D. E., Rønnestad, M. H., and Willutzki, U. (2004), "Fifty years of process-outcome research: Continuity and change," in A. E. Bergin and S. L. Garfield (eds), *Handbook of Psychotherapy and Behavior Change*, 4th edn, pp. 307–90 (New York, NY: Wiley).

Robles, T. (1990), *A Concert for Four Hemispheres in Psychotherapy* (New York, NY: Vantage Press).

Rogers, C. (1961), *On Becoming a Person* (Boston, MA: Houghton Mifflin).

Rosen, S. (1982), *My Voice will go With You: The Teaching Tales of Milton H. Erickson* (New York, NY: W. W. Norton & Co.).

Rosenthal, R., and Jacobson, L. (1968), *Pygmalion in the Classroom* (New York, NY: Holt, Rinehart & Winston).

Rossi, E. L. (1973), "Psychological Shocks and Creative Moments in Psychotherapy," *American Journal of Clinical Hypnosis*, 16, pp. 9–22.

Rossi, E. L. (2004), "Milton H. Erickson: The Cheerful Work Ethic of an American Farm Boy," *Milton H Erickson Foundation Newsletter*, 24, 3 (Phoenix, AZ: Milton H. Erickson Foundation Archives), p. 9.

Sanghavi, D. (2003), *A Map of the Child: A Pediatrician's Tour of the Body* (New York, NY: Henry Holt).

Selvini, M. (1988), *The Work of Mara Selvini Palazzoli*, ed. Matteo Selvini (New Jersey: Jason Aronson).

Shapiro, E. S., and Kratochwill, T. R. (1988), *Behavioral Assessment in Schools* (New York, NY: Gildford).

Short, D. (1999), "Hypnosis and Children: An Analysis of Theory and Research," in B. Matthews and J. Edgette (eds), *Current Thinking and Practices in Brief Therapy* (Philadelphia: Taylor and Francis) pp. 285–335.

Short, D. (2001), "Mandatory counseling: Helping those who do not want to be helped," in B. Geary, and J. K. Zeig (eds), *The Handbook of Ericksonian Psychotherapy* (Phoenix, AZ: Milton H. Erickson Foundation Press) pp. 333–51.

Snyder, C. R. (ed.) (2000), *Handbook of Hope: Theory, Measures, and Applications* (New York, NY: Academic Press).

Spanos, N. P., and Gorassini, D. R. (1984), "Structure of hypnotic test suggestions and attributes of responding involuntarily," *Journal of Personality and Social Psychology*, 46, 3, pp. 688–96.

Thomsen, J., et al. (1983), "Placebo effect in surgery for Méniere's disease: Three-year follow-up," *Otolaryngology—Head and Neck Surgery*, 91, pp. 183–6.

Volgyesi, F. A. (1954), "School for patients: hypnosis-therapy and psycho-prophylaxis," *British Journal of Medical Hypnotism*, 5, pp. 8–17.

Wampold, B. E. (2001), *The Great Psychotherapy Debate: Models, methods, and Findings*. (Hillsdale, NJ: Erlbaum).

Wann, D. L., and Branscombe, N. R. (1990), "Person perception when aggressive or nonaggressive sports are primed," *Aggressive Behavior*, 16, pp. 27–32.

Waters, D. B., and Lawrence, E. C. (1993), *Competence, Courage, and Change: An Approach to Family Therapy* (New York, NY: W. W. Norton & Co.).

Watzlawick, P. (1978), *The Language of Change: Elements of Therapeutic Communication* (New York, NY: Basic Books).

Watzlawick, P., Weakland, J., and Fisch, R. (1974), *Change: Principles of Problem Formation and Problem Resolution* (New York, NY: W. W. Norton & Co.).

Weinberger, J. (1994), "Conclusion: Can personality change?," in T. F. Heatherton and J. Weinberger (eds), *Can Personality Change?* (Washington, DC: American Psychological Association), pp. 333–50.

Weinberger, J. (1995), "Common factors aren't so common: The common factors dilemma," *Clinical Psychology: Science and Practice*, 2, pp. 45–69.

Weitzenhoffer, A. M. (1989), *The Practice of Hypnotism*, Vol. I (New York, NY: John Wiley & Sons).

White, M. (1988), "The Externalizing of the Problem and the Re-authoring of Lives and Relationships," *Dulwich Centre Newsletter*, Summer.

Wilson, R. R. (2001), "Anxiety Disorders," in B. Geary and J. K. Zeig (eds), *The Handbook of Ericksonian Psychotherapy* (Phoenix, AZ: Milton H. Erickson Foundation Press) pp. 215–29.

Wolpe, J. (1969), *The Practice of Behavior Therapy* (New York, NY: Pergamon Press).

Yapko, M. D. (2003), *Trancework: An Introduction to the Practice of Clinical Hypnosis*, 3rd edn, (New York, NY: Brunner-Routledge).

Zajonc, R. B., and Markus, H. (1982), "Affective and cognitive factors in preferences," *Journal of Consumer Research*, *9*, pp. 123–31.

Zeig, J. K. (1980), *A Teaching Seminar with Milton H. Erickson* (New York, NY: Bruner/Mazel).

Zeig, J. K. (1985), *Experiencing Erickson: An Introduction to the Man and his Work* (New York, NY: Brunner/Mazel).

Zeig, J. K. (1992), "The virtues of our faults: A key concept of Ericksonian therapy," in J. K. Zeig (ed.), *The Evolution of Psychotherapy: The Second Conference* (New York, NY: Brunner/Mazel) pp. 252–66.

Zeig, J. K., and Geary, B. B. (1990), "Seeds of Strategic and Interactional Psychotherapies: Seminal Contributions of Milton H. Erickson," *American Journal of Clinical Hypnosis*, *33*, 2, pp. 105–12.

Index

reframing 161–7, 218, 219
refusal 193, 205–6
regression 177–8, 181
rehearsal technique 178
reorientation 35, 104, 153–84
resistance, passive 141
resources, untapped 234
rituals 45, 110, 112, 148
Robles, T. 82
Rogers, C. 174
Rosen, S. 54
Rosenthal, R. 150
Rossi, E. L. 48, 70, 71, 122, 146, 148, 198, 200
Rossi, S. I. 48, 70, 71, 122, 146, 148, 198, 200
Rothovius, A. E. 10, 112, 113, 122

Sanghavi, D. 106
Satir, V. 174
scarring 111
schizophrenia 201n
Sector, I. I. 118, 130, 210
seeding 101, 102
self-
    anchored scaling 104
    assessment 64
    destructive behavior 190
    fulfilling prophecy 43, 51, 150
    hypnosis 136
    identity 74
    image 191, 209, 224
    observation 173
    punishment 203
Selvini, M. 214
sexual abuse 127, 224
shame 137, 164, 186, 215
Shapiro, E. S. 73
shock, anaphylactic 68
Short, D. 35, 61, 73, 76, 102, 112, 118, 119, 144, 149, 165–6, 183, 186, 200, 216, 219, 220, 222
sleep deprivation 27
smoking 157, 190
Snyder, C. R. 114
Socrates 100
solution-focused therapy 60, 104, 180
Spanos, N. P. 121
splitting, prognostic 63
stimuli:
    ambiguous 131
    noxious 90
    painful 121
    unnerving 53
stuttering 43

suggestion:
    contradictory 143
    contraindications for 223
    indirect 122
    permissive 129
    waking 149
suicidal ideations 176
suspense 48
symptom:
    definition 59
    displacement 211–12
    embellishment 211, 213
    prescription 36, 209
    scheduling 211
    substitution 211–12

tachycardia 15
teleology 29
temporal relations 177
therapeutic agenda 211
Thomsen, J. 114
thought and action, separation of 42
time distortion 103, 177, 179
Tonsager, M. E. 62
Tour de France 11
trauma, childhood 52, 93
treatment:
    outcome 70
    plan 66, 190

ulcers 30, 113
unconscious mind 27, 31, 69–72, 103, 130, 232
utilization 234–5

vicious cycle 43, 56, 216
Volgyesi, F. A. 30, 114

Wann, D. L. 101
warts 118–19
Waters, D. B. 114
Watzlawick, P. 162, 201
Weinberger, J. 131
Weitzenhoffer, A. M. 112
White, M. 173
Wilson, R. R. 58
witch doctors 136–7
Wolpe, J. 90
words, double meaning of 143

Yapko, M. D. 74, 84

Zajonc, R. B. 125, 137
Zanna, M. P. 23
Zeig, J. K. 11, 92, 115, 123, 148, 186, 213, 214, 220, 221

.

CPSIA information can be obtained
at www.ICGtesting.com
Printed in the USA
LVHW081819250722
724363LV00004B/118